Multiple Choice Question
in Ophthalmic and Neur

Also available

MCQs in Ophthalmology
Anthony Vivian and Ruth Manners

Multiple Choice Questions in Ophthalmic and Neuroanatomy

O.J. LEHMANN
MA (Cantab), BM BCh (Oxon)
Moorfields Eye Hospital, London

Formerly Anatomy Demonstrator, Manchester University, and Senior House Officer, Manchester Royal Eye Hospital

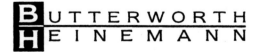

Butterworth-Heinemann Ltd
Linacre House, Jordan Hill, Oxford OX2 8DP

⦵ A member of the Reed Elsevier group

OXFORD   LONDON   BOSTON
MUNICH   NEW DELHI   SINGAPORE   SYDNEY
TOKYO   TORONTO   WELLINGTON

First published 1993

© Butterworth-Heinemann Ltd 1993

British Library Cataloguing in Publication Data
Lehmann, O. J.
   Multiple Choice Questions in Ophthalmic
   and Neuroanatomy
   I. Title
   612.8

ISBN 0 7506 0988 5

Typeset by TecSet Ltd, Wallington, Surrey
Printed and bound in Great Britain by Biddles Ltd, Guildford
& Kings Lynn

Contents

Preface

I wrote these questions from notes that I made while preparing for the College of Ophthalmologists' primary examination. At the time it was difficult to gauge the standard expected as there were no questions available. I hope this book proves helpful to the many candidates who need to learn this sort of anatomy and trust its appeal extends beyond budding ophthalmologists and general surgeons to include optometrists and orthoptists.

I have tried hard to minimize any ambiguity in the questions and am most grateful to Ian Simmonds, Sundeep Kheterpal, Sheila Kelleher and Andrew Morris for their very helpful comments and suggestions. Finally I would like to thank those friends and colleagues who have encouraged me both to write this book and to pursue a career in ophthalmology.

O.J. Lehmann

Abbreviations

The following abbreviations are used in the text:
- I Olfactory nerve
- II Optic nerve
- III Oculomotor nerve
- IV Trochlear nerve
- V Trigeminal nerve (V_1 ophthalmic, V_2 maxillary and V_3 mandibular divisions of the trigeminal nerve)
- VI Abducent nerve
- VIII Facial nerve
- VIII Vestibulocochlear nerve
- IX Glossopharyngeal nerve
- X Vagus nerve
- XI Accessory nerve
- XII Hypoglossal nerve

1 Osteology

1 Which of the following statements is/are correct?
   A   The anterior fontanelle closes before the posterior
   B   The metopic suture lies between unfused frontal bones
   C   The pterion is the site of articulation of four bones including the parietal and zygomatic bones
   D   A spine of bone lies inferior to the piriform aperture
   E   Embryologically the orbital roof is derived from mesoderm

2 The sphenoid bone
   A   Articulates with the occipital bone
   B   Forms most of the middle cranial fossa floor
   C   Has two wings separated by the inferior orbital fissure
   D   Is grooved by the internal carotid artery
   E   Has its overlying dura innervated by nervus spinosus

Osteology: Answers

1   A False
    B True
    C False
    D True
    E True
The anterior fontanelle closes at ≈18 months, with the posterior closing at 6–9 months. The metopic suture lies between the unfused halves of the frontal bone. It disappears once fusion occurs, generally by the age of 7, although the suture may persist in up to 7% of the population. The pterion is the site where the frontal, parietal and temporal bones, as well as the greater wing of the sphenoid, lie adjacent to each other. It is crossed by the anterior branch of the middle meningeal artery. The anterior nasal (piriform) aperture lies above the anterior nasal spine which is formed by both maxillae. All the orbital 'walls' are derived from mesoderm.

2   A True
    B True
    C False
    D True
    E True
The basiocciput and basisphenoid fuse by ≈25 years of age. The sphenoid bone has two greater and two lesser wings which are separated on each side by the superior orbital fissure. The nervus spinosus is the meningeal branch of the mandibular nerve. It crosses the foramen spinosum with the middle meningeal artery and mainly supplies the dura of the middle cranial fossa.

3 **The following form the walls (including the roof and floor) of the pterygopalatine fossa**
   A   Lesser wing of sphenoid
   B   Greater wing of sphenoid
   C   Pterygoid process of sphenoid
   D   Perpendicular plate of ethmoid
   E   Maxilla

4 **Which of the following statements is/are correct?**
   A   The orbit is pyramidal in shape
   B   The medial orbital walls are parallel
   C   The zygomatic nerve divides within the temporal bone to form two branches
   D   The ethmoidal foramina lie along the fronto-ethmoidal suture
   E   The optic canal lies above the level of the ethmoidal foramina

5 **The paranasal sinuses**
   A   Consist of four main pairs of sinuses
   B   Are all present at term
   C   Include one that may extend into the lesser wing of the sphenoid
   D   May indent the lateral nasal wall
   E   May include a small sinus in the palatine bone

3 A False
   B True
   C True
   D False
   E True
The boundaries of the pterygopalatine fossa are:
Anteriorly – posterior surface of maxilla
Posteriorly – pterygoid process and greater wing of sphenoid
Medially   – perpendicular plate of palatine bone
Laterally   – fossa communicates with infratemporal fossa

4 A True
   B True
   C False
   D True
   E False
The orbit is a quadrilateral pyramid with parallel medial walls. Its ethmoid component articulates with the frontal bone (i.e. the orbital roof) at the fronto-ethmoidal suture, along which the ethmoidal foramina lie. The optic canal therefore lies below this level. The zygomatic nerve runs in a groove and canal in the lateral orbital wall, dividing within the orbit or the zygomatic bone to form zygomaticofacial and zygomaticotemporal branches.

5 A True
   B False
   C True
   D True
   E True
There are four paired sinuses: the frontal, maxillary, ethmoid and sphenoid sinuses. These sinuses are poorly developed at term, with the frontal sinus, in particular, being absent. The sphenoid sinus may extend into both sphenoidal wings and partially (or completely) encircle the optic nerve. The bulla ethmoidalis, formed by middle ethmoidal air cells, indents the lateral nasal wall. The palatine bone often contains a sinus in its orbital process.

6 Which of these structures enter the jugular foramen?
   A   Superior petrosal sinus
   B   Sigmoid sinus
   C   VIII
   D   IX
   E   X

7 Emissary veins pass through the following foramina
   A   Parietal foramen
   B   Foramen lacerum
   C   Foramen caecum
   D   Foramen rotundum
   E   Foramen ovale

8 Named nerves pass through the following bones
   A   Parietal
   B   Occipital
   C   Petrous temporal
   D   Palatine
   E   Maxilla

6 A False
   B True
   C False
   D True
   E True

The superior petrosal sinus drains into the transverse sinus, which becomes the sigmoid sinus. This drains into the superior bulb of the internal jugular vein which also drains the inferior petrosal sinus. The internal jugular vein, IX, X and XI all traverse the jugular foramen.

7 A True
   B True
   C True
   D False
   E True

Emissary veins cross the skull to connect the venous sinuses with external veins. The parietal emissary veins connect the superior sagittal sinus with the scalp veins. Other veins connect the cavernous sinus with the pterygopalatine plexus via the foramina lacerum, ovale and that of Vesalius. Rarely a vein may connect nasal veins with the superior sagittal sinus via the foramen caecum.

8 A False
   B True
   C True
   D True
   E True
   In A None
   In B Spinal root of XI, and XII
   In C VII
   In D Greater and lesser palatine nerves
   In E Infraorbital

9 The following transmit both neural and vascular structures
- A Optic canal
- B Carotid canal
- C Jugular foramen
- D Foramen spinosum
- E Stylomastoid foramen

10 Which of the following statements regarding the external nose is/are correct?
- A Inferiorly its skeleton is entirely composed of cartilage
- B Laterally it contains the turbinate bones
- C It is divided into equal halves by the nasal septum
- D It contains an anteriorly projecting spine of bone
- E It possesses a single vomeronasal organ

9 A True
   B True
   C True
   D True
   E True
  In **A** Optic nerve and ophthalmic artery
  In **B** Sympathetic nerve fibres and internal carotid artery
  In **C** IX, X and XI, internal jugular vein and inferior petrosal sinus
  In **D** Meningeal branch of the mandibular nerve and middle meningeal artery
  In **E** VII and stylomastoid branch of the posterior auricular artery

10 A True
   B False
   C False
   D True
   E False
The nose consists of two parts – the external nose and the nasal cavity. The external nose's skeleton consists of the two nasal bones superiorly with the lateral and greater nasal cartilages inferiorly. The nasal cavity is divided into two halves by the nasal septum, and it (and not the external nose) contains the turbinate bones in its lateral walls. The anterior nasal spine, formed from both maxillae, lies in the external nose and forms the inferior boundary of the anterior nasal aperture. The vomeronasal organs are vestigial olfactory structures lying on either side of the septum.

11   The following bones form part of the orbital margin
  A   Ethmoid
  B   Lacrimal
  C   Zygomatic
  D   Lesser wing of the sphenoid
  E   Maxilla

12   The orbital roof
  A   Is partly formed by the greater wing of the sphenoid
  B   Articulates with the lesser wing of the sphenoid
  C   May be invaded by the ethmoid sinus
  D   May contain part of the frontal sinus
  E   Articulates with the ethmoid

13   The orbital floor
  A   Contains the pterygoid process of the palatine bone
  B   Receives a contribution from the maxilla
  C   Is easily damaged in 'blow-out' fractures as it is the thinnest orbital wall
  D   Contains a groove that transmits a branch of the ophthalmic artery
  E   Is separated from the greater wing of the sphenoid by the sphenomaxillary fissure

11 A False
    B True
    C True
    D False
    E True
The orbital margin is formed by the following bones:
Supraorbital margin – frontal bone
Lateral margin   – zygomatic process of frontal bone and frontal
                        process of zygomatic bone
Infraorbital margin – zygomatic bone laterally, maxilla medially
Medial margin   – anterior lacrimal crest of maxilla
                        – posterior lacrimal crest of lacrimal bone

12 A False
    B False
    C True
    D True
    E True
The triangular-shaped orbital roof is formed by the orbital plate of
the frontal bone with a contribution from the lesser wing of the
sphenoid. The roof articulates with the ethmoid bone at the fronto-
ethmoidal suture and may not be invaded by the frontal and
ethmoidal sinuses. Rarely the sphenoid sinus may encircle the optic
nerve, thus invading the sphenoid's lesser wing and posing a danger
to sight in trans-sphenoidal pituitary surgery.

13 A False
    B True
    C False
    D False
    E True
The infraorbital artery and nerve groove the orbital floor, which is
formed by three bones: the maxilla, the zyogmatic and the orbital
process of the Palatine bone. The infraorbital is a branch of the third
part of the maxillary artery. The sphenomaxillary fissure is better
known as the inferior orbital fissure. The orbital plate of the ethmoid
(lamina paparycea) is thinner than the floor.

14 The medial orbital wall receives contributions from the
  A Orbital plate of the ethmoid
  B Lesser wing of the sphenoid
  C Frontal bone
  D Lacrimal bone
  E Maxilla

15 The lateral orbital wall
  A Contains a fossa for the lacrimal gland
  B Forms part of the origin of lateral rectus
  C In part lies medial to the temporal lobe
  D Has its middle third formed by part of the zygomatic bone
  E Is closely related to the temporal fossa

16 Which of the following statements is/are correct?
  A The lacrimal sac lies posterior to the lacrimal crest of the lacrimal bone
  B The aponeurosis of levator palpabrae superioris attaches to the marginal tubercle (of Whitnall)
  C The optic foramen lies at the orbital apex
  D The annulus of Zinn (common tendinous ring) bridges both orbital fissures
  E Both orbital fissues are partially closed by muscle or fibrous tissue

14 A True
B False
C False
D True
E True
The medial orbital wall consists of four bones
Frontal process of maxilla ⎫ Anteriorly
Lacrimal bone ⎪
Orbital plate of ethmoid ⎬ to
Part of body of sphenoid ⎭ posteriorly

15 A False
B True
C True
D False
E True
The lacrimal gland indents the orbital roof. The zygomatic bone forms the anterior third, and the greater wing of the sphenoid the posterior two-thirds, of the lateral orbital wall. This wall separates the orbit from both the middle cranial and temporal fossae and has a spine to which lateral rectus attaches.

16 A False
B True
C False
D False
E True
The lacrimal crests bound the lacrimal fossa in which the lacrimal sac lies. They are formed from part of the frontal process of the maxilla anteriorly and the lacrimal bone posteriorly. The optic foramen lies anteromedial to the orbital apex. The annulus of Zinn does not bridge the inferior orbital fissure, which like its fellow is closed by fibrous tissue.

17 The orbital periosteum (periorbita)

A   Is tightly attached to the orbital walls
B   Forms the orbital septa
C   Forms the common tendinous ring
D   Anchors the trochlea 8 mm behind the orbital margin
E   Is continuous with the periosteum of the frontal bone

18 The adult orbit of a female differs from that of a male in having

A   Less prominent supraciliary ridges
B   Smaller constituent bones
C   Smoother orbital walls
D   Its widest diameter posterior to the orbital rim
E   Some of the above-mentioned features occurring prior to puberty

17 A False
    B True
    C True
    D False
    E True

The orbital periosteum is loosely attached to the bones of the orbit except at certain points, including suture lines, foramina and the orbital margin. It is continuous with the periosteum of the bones surrounding the orbit and in addition forms the orbital septum and common tendinous ring. The trochlea's attachment to the under-surface of the frontal bone is ≈ 4 mm behind the orbital margin.

18 A True
    B False
    C True
    D False
    E False

Before puberty there is little difference between the orbits of the two sexes. After puberty the female orbit is more elongated than the male with rounder, smoother bones and smaller superciliary ridges. All orbits are widest some 1.5 cm posterior to the orbital margin.

2 Anatomy of the head and neck

1 **The mandible**
- A Consists of two halves which unite by two years of age
- B Has a condylar process which articulates with the cartilage lining the mandibular fossa
- C Has a foramen below the second molar tooth through which branches of the inferior alveolar nerve emerge
- D Is connected to the sphenoid bone
- E Is indented by salivary glands

2 **Regarding the dentition**
- A The deciduous teeth are shed at 6–12 years
- B The permanent teeth erupt by 18 years
- C The premolars have four cusps
- D The mandibular molars have five cusps
- E Enamel covers the whole tooth

Anatomy of the head and neck: answers

1   A   True
      B   False
      C   False
      D   True
      E   True

The two halves of the mandible meet at the symphysis menti, with fusion occurring at about 2 years. The condylar process of the mandible articulates with a cartilaginous articular disc that divides the temporomandibular joint space into two. Branches of the inferior alveolar nerve emerge from the mental foramen, below the second premolar tooth. The sphenomandibular ligament connects the lingula of the mandible with the sphenoid bone. The sublingual and submandibular fossae, which contain two salivary glands, lie on either side of the mylohyoid line.

2   A   True
      B   False
      C   False
      D   True
      E   False

Deciduous or milk teeth are shed at 6–12 years as many of the permanent teeth erupt. The third permanent molars (wisdom teeth) emerge from 18 years of age onwards. Premolars are bicuspid, whereas the maxillary molars have four cusps and the mandibular molars five. Enamel covers the crown of the tooth, whereas the root is covered by cementum.

3 The parotid gland

  A Lies in direct contact with subcutaneous tissue

  B Is traversed by the retromandibular vein

  C Is traversed by the upper division of VII passing above the zygomatic arch

  D Receives fibres from the inferior salivatory nucleus of IX

  E Contains lymph nodes to which orbital structures drain

4 The following are innervated by a nerve passing through the foramen ovale

  A Masseter

  B Posterior belly of digastric

  C Stylohyoid

  D Mylohyoid

  E Tensor veli palatini

3 A False
B True
C False
D True
E True

The parotid gland is enclosed by a capsule and lies below the zygomatic arch. Traversing the gland are the retromandibular vein, VII and external carotid artery. The gland is supplied by parasympathetic fibres from the otic ganglion whose preganglionic neurons arise from the inferior salivatory nucleus of IX. Laterally placed orbital structures drain to the pre-auricular lymph nodes.

4 A True
B False
C False
D True
E True

V_3 crosses the foramen ovale and supplies the muscles of mastication, including masseter as well as mylohyoid and tensor veli palatini. The latter is the only muscle of the soft palate to be supplied by V_3, the remainder being supplied by the cranial root of XI conveyed to the pharyngeal plexus by X. The posterior belly of digastric is derived from the second pharyngeal arch (as is stylohyoid), and both are thus supplied by the nerve of that arch (VII).

5 Which of the following statements is/are correct?
   A Taste is conveyed by fibres of VII, IX and X
   B XII supplies all the lingual muscles
   C The tongue's position is changed by the intrinsic lingual muscles
   D The fifth branch of the external carotid is the main arterial supply to the tongue
   E XII conveys fibres to sternohyoid and omohyoid

6 The following receive fibres from the trigeminal nerve
   A Buccinator
   B Anterior belly of digastric
   C Stapedius
   D Tympanic membrane
   E Orbicularis oculi

5 A True
   B False
   C False
   D False
   E True

Taste is conveyed by the chorda tympani fibres (of VII) from the anterior two-thirds of the tongue, by IX from the posterior third and by X from a small part of the valleculae. All muscles of the tongue, except palatoglossus, are supplied by XII, palatoglossus being supplied by the pharyngeal plexus. The extrinsic muscles change the position of the tongue, whereas the intrinsic muscles mainly alter its shape. The lingual artery, the main arterial supply to the tongue, is the third branch of the external carotid. The hypoglossal nerve conveys fibres from C1 and C2 which form the upper root of the ansa cervicalis and supply sternohyoid and omohyoid.

6 A True
   B True
   C False
   D True
   E True

Although the muscles of facial expression receive their motor supply from VII, their proprioceptive innervation is derived from the nerve supplying the overlying skin. Therefore, both orbicularis oculi and buccinator have a sensory supply from V. The anterior belly of diagastric is a first-arch derivative and is thus supplied by the nerve of the first arch (V). Stapedius is a second-arch derivative and is supplied by the nerve of the second arch (VII). The tympanic membrane is supplied by the auriculotemporal nerve (branch of V_3) as well as by VII, IX and X.

7 The following are innervated by a nerve traversing part of the temporal bone
  A Tensor tympani
  B Stylohyoid
  C Buccinator
  D Submandibular ganglion
  E Occipitalis

8 Which of the following statements about the scalp is/are correct?
  A Occipitalis and frontalis are both innervated by the facial nerve
  B Frontalis attaches to orbicularis oculi
  C Occipitalis attaches to the superior nuchal line
  D A potential subaponeurotic space extends to lie anterior to part of the cornea
  E It is a site of anastomosis between branches of the external and internal carotid arteries

7 A False
   B True
   C True
   D True
   E True

Tensor tympani is supplied by the nerve to medial pterygoid. This is a branch of V_3 which crosses the foramen ovale in the greater wing of the sphenoid. All the remaining structures are supplied by VII, which traverses the petrous temporal bone, with the submandibular ganglion being supplied by its chorda tympani branch.

8 A True
   B True
   C False
   D True
   E True

Occipitalis and frontalis each consist of two bellies inserting into the galea aponeurotica, and are innervated by the posterior auricular and temporal branches of VII, respectively. Occipitalis attaches to the lateral two-thirds of the highest nuchal line, whereas frontalis which has no bony attachments attaches to muscle, including orbicularis oculi. A potential subaponeurotic space exists beneath the galea, extending under orbicularis oculi into the eyelids. Hence subgaleal haemorrhage may cause periorbital ecchymoses. The scalp has a rich vascular supply, with two branches from the internal carotid (supraorbital and supratrochlear) anastomosing with three branches from the external carotid (occipital, posterior auricular and superficial temporal).

9 Which of the following statements about lymphatic drainage of the head and neck is/are correct?

A   Lymph from this area drains to the deep cervical nodes surrounding the internal jugular vein

B   On the left side of the deep cervical nodes drain directly into the thoracic duct

C   The submental lymph nodes form part of the inner circle of nodes

D   Superficial lymphatics generally accompany arteries

E   Medially placed ocular structures drain to the sublingual nodes

10 The skin of the nose is supplied by branches of the following

A   Ophthalmic artery

B   Anterior ethmoidal artery and nerve

C   Infraorbital artery

D   Infratrochlear nerve

E   Facial artery

9 A True
   B False
   C False
   D False
   E False

Lymph from the head and neck drains via inner and outer circles of nodes to deep cervical nodes and then to the jugular lymph trunk. This drains to the thoracic duct on the left or the internal jugular and brachiocephalic veins on the right. Superficial lymphatics generally accompany veins, whereas deeper ones follow arteries. Submental lymph nodes form part of the outer circle of nodes, while the inner circle surrounds the trachea and oesophagus. (It consists of pretracheal, paratracheal and retropharyngeal nodes.)

10 A True
   B True
   C False
   D True
   E True

The branches of the ophthalmic artery supplying nasal skin include the dorsal nasal and anterior ethmoidal arteries (branches of the latter's nerve also supply the skin as the external nasal nerve). The infratrochlear nerve, a branch of the nasociliary, supplies some nasal skin, as does the angular artery, the terminal part of the facial artery. The infraorbital artery emerges from the infraorbital foramen and supplies adjacent facial tissues, giving orbital branches to inferior rectus and inferior oblique, but no nasal branches.

11 Which of the following statements is/are correct?

A The epithelium lining the nasal septum is unciliated

B Lymph from the nasal cavity drains to the sublingual and paratracheal nodes

C The vomer articulates with the nasal bones

D Nasal veins may communicate with cerebral venous sinuses

E The middle concha is the largest turbinate bone

12 Regarding the nasal conchae

A They are united anteriorly

B The spheno-ethmoidal recess opens into the superior meatus

C The maxillary sinus drains into the middle meatus

D The nasolacrimal duct enters the inferior meatus 2 cm behind the anterior nares

E Air cells may indent the lateral wall of the nose

11 A False
   B False
   C False
   D True
   E False

The nasal septum, lined by a respiratory-type mucous membrane, consists of a ciliated columnar epithelium. Lymph from the anterior half of the nose drains to the submandibular nodes, whereas that from the posterior part passes to the retropharyngeal and deep cervical nodes. The vomer has no articulation with the two nasal bones. Approximately 1% of patients have a patent foramen caecum joining the nasal veins with the superior sagittal sinus. The inferior concha is the largest of the three turbinate bones.

12 A False
   B False
   C True
   D True
   E True

Only the upper and middle conchae (turbinate bones) are united anteriorly. The sphenoethmoidal recess, into which the sphenoidal sinus drains, lies above the superior concha. The superior meatus lies below it and drains the posterior ethmoidal air cells. The nasolacrimal duct drains into the inferior meatus, whereas the other paranasal sinuses drain to the middle meatus. The middle ethmoidal air cells form the bulla ethmoidalis, a bulge on the lateral nasal wall.

13 **The Eustachian tube**
    A   Is cartilaginous throughout its length
    B   Connects the pharynx with the mastoid air cells
    C   Has its pharyngeal opening occluded by a fold of mucous.
        membrane
    D   In adults opens at the level of the hard palate
    E   Lies adjacent to salpingopharyngeus

14 **The palatine tonsils**
    A   Lie above the opening of the Eustachian tube
    B   Lie between the palatoglossal and palatopharyngeal arches
    C   Lie in a fossa bed formed by palatoglossus
    D   May contain a cleft
    E   Are supplied by a branch of the facial artery

15 **The auricle is innervated by branches from the following**
    A V_2
    B V_3
    C   VII
    D   X
    E   Ventral rami of C2 and C3

13 A False
   B True
   C True
   D False
   E True
The Eustachian tube is approximately 3 cm long, and has an osseous lateral third with a cartilaginous medial two-thirds. It connects the nasopharynx with the mastoid air cells. Its pharyngeal end lies just below the skull base and is occluded by folds of mucous membrane. It lies adjacent to salpingopharyngeus which inserts into part of the Eustachian tube.

14 A False
   B True
   C False
   D True
   E True
The palatine tonsils lie in the tonsilar fossa between the palatoglossal and palatopharyngeal arches, several centimetres below the opening of the Eustachian tube. The floor of the fossa is formed by superior constrictor, and the intratonsilar cleft extends into the upper part of the tonsil. The tonsils have a rich vascular supply derived mainly from the tonsilar branch of the facial artery, with contributions from the ascending pharyngeal, ascending palatine and lingual vessels.

15 A False
   B True
   C True
   D True
   E True
The auricle or pinna consists of a cartilaginous framework covered by skin. It is innervated by the:
Auriculotemporal nerve (V_3)
Auricular branches of VII and X
Lesser occipital nerve (C2)
Greater auricular nerve (C2 and C3)

16 The tympanic membrane
- A Lies vertically in the external acoustic meatus
- B Has the pars tensa lying superiorly
- C Articulates with the handle of the malleus
- D Is attached to tensor tympani
- E Is innervated by IX

17 Regarding the inner ear
- A The scala vestubili contains endolymph
- B The scalae vestibuli and tympani are connected
- C The scala vestibuli lies next to the round window
- D The posterior semicircular canal indents the petrous temporal bone
- E Endolymph passes to the posterior cranial fossa

16 A False
   B False
   C True
   D False
   E True

The tympanic membrane lies at an angle of 55° to the floor of the external acoustic meatus. It consists of two parts: a small pars flaccida superiorly and the larger pars tensa below. The handle of the malleus forms a small depression in the tympanic membrane, the centre of which is called the umbo. Tensor tympani arises from the Eustachian tube and inserts into the handle of the malleus. The tympanic membrane is innervated by: the auriculotemporal nerve, the tympanic branch of IX, the auricular branch of X as well as possibly by branches of VII.

17 A False
   B True
   C False
   D False
   E True

The scalae vestibuli and tympani are filled with perilymph and lie on either side of the cochlear duct, communicating with one another via the helicotrema. The ends of the two scalae are closed by the fenestra vestibuli (oval window) and fenestra tympani (round window), respectively. The anterior semicircular canal lies above the other two and forms the arcuate eminence on the petrous temporal bone. Endolymph from the inner ear passes via the endolymphatic duct to the endolymphatic sac, which lies in the posterior cranial fossa.

18 Which of the following statements is/are correct?

  A VII contains parasympathetic fibres as it emerges from the stylomastoid foramen

  B The mastoid air cells communicate with the nasopharynx

  C The entrance to the mastoid antrum lies above the tympanic membrane

  D The muscles of the middle ear are all innervated by VII

  E The semicircular canals have equal numbers of ampullated and non-ampullated ends

19 The pterygopalatine fossa communicates with the

  A Orbit

  B Nasal cavity

  C Oral cavity

  D Infratemporal fossa

  E Foramen lacerum

18 A False
B True
C True
D False
E False

VII emerges from the stylomastoid foramen containing just motor fibres. The parasympathetic fibres of N. intermedius leave VII in the chorda tympani. The mastoid antrum, a large sinus in the temporal bone, communicates with the other air cells and opens into the epitympanic recess above the tympanic membrane. This enables the mastoid air cells to communicate with the nasopharynx via the Eustachian tube. Only stapedius is innervated by VII, as tensor tympani is supplied by the nerve to medial pterygoid (V_3). The non-ampullated ends of the posterior and lateral semicircular canals are fused, so that in total there are three ampullated and two non-ampullated ends.

19 A True
B True
C True
D True
E True

The pterygopalatine fossa lies below the orbital apex between the posterior surface of the maxilla and the anterior surface of the pterygoid process of the sphenoid. It communicates with: the orbit via the inferior orbital fissure, the nasal cavity via the sphenopalatine foramen, the infratemporal fossa via the pterygomaxillary fissure, the foramen lacerum via the pterygoid canal, and the oral cavity via the greater palatine canal.

20 The contents of the pterygopalatine fossa include the
   A   Second part of the maxillary artery
   B   Maxillary nerve
   C   Sphenopalatine ganglion
   D   Pterygoid venous plexus
   E   Nervus intermedius

21 Which of the following statements about the cervical vertebrae is/are correct?
   A   They all have a foramen in their transverse processes
   B   The sixth vertebra has the longest spinous process
   C   The atlas has a small body
   D   Rotatory movement occurs at the atlanto-occipital joints
   E   The transverse ligament limits lateral rotation between the atlas and odontoid peg

22 The spinal cord
   A   Widens above the level of T1
   B   Contains a central mass of white matter
   C   Has fibres conveying kinaesthesia from the lumbosacral area, located laterally
   D   Is directly attached to its spinal nerves
   E   Receives a major vascular supply from radicular arteries

20 A False
B True
C True
D False
E False

The main contents of the fossa are the pterygopalatine ganglion, V_3 and branches of the third part of the maxillary artery (this artery is divided into three parts by the lateral pterygoid muscle and these parts lie before, on and distal to the muscle, respectively).

21 A True
B False
C False
D False
E False

All the cervical vertebrae have foramina transversaria with the vertebral artery passing through the foramina of C1–C6. The atlas vertebra has no body, whereas C7 (vertebra prominens) has the longest spinous process. All rotatory movements occur between the atlas (C1) and the axis (C2), the transverse ligament preventing posterior dislocation of the odontoid peg.

22 A True
B False
C False
D False
E True

The spinal cord has cervical and lumbosacral enlargements for the brachial and lumbosacral plexuses. Centrally the cord consists of a mass of grey matter surrounded by myelinated fibres (white matter) peripherally. Kinaesthetic fibres from the lumbosacral area lie medially in the dorsal columns (running in the gracile tracts). Only the anterior and posterior nerve roots are attached to the cord and fuse to form spinal nerves in the intervertebral foramina. Although supplied by the anterior and posterior spinal arteries, the cord receives a significant vascular supply from the radicular arteries.

23   The anterior triangle of the neck contains
  A   The strap muscles
  B   Both bellies of digastric
  C   The inferior belly of omohyoid
  D   The carotid sinus
  E   The carotid body

24   The posterior triangle of the neck
  A   Is bounded anteriorly by trapezius
  B   Has the vagus nerve crossing its floor
  C   Is roofed by investing fascia
  D   Contains the external jugular vein
  E   Is crossed by the second part of the subclavian artery

25   The following structures lie within the carotid sheath
  A   Internal jugular vein
  B   Jugulo-omohyoid lymph node
  C   Jugulo-digastric lymph node
  D   Vagus nerve
  E   Carotid body

23 A True
  B True
  C False
  D True
  E True

The anterior triangle of the neck lies between sternocleidomastoid, the midline and the lower border of the mandible. It contains the strap muscles, which include both bellies of digastric, as well as the common carotid artery and its bifurcation. The carotid sinus lies at the bifurcation, with the carotid body lying adjacent to it. The inferior belly of omohyoid lies outside the anterior triangle and runs from the upper border of the scapula to its tendon's attachment to the clavicle.

24 A False
  B False
  C True
  D True
  E False

The posterior triangle of the neck lies between sternocleidomastoid anteriorly, trapezius posteriorly and the clavicle. The accessory nerve supplies sternocleidomastoid as it passes through it, before crossing the floor of the posterior triangle to supply trapezius as well. The third part of the subclavian artery (the portion formed after it has passed under scalenus anterior) lies in the posterior triangle.

25 A True
  B True
  C True
  D True
  E True

All the structures listed lie within the carotid sheath, as does the ansa cervicalis. The latter is formed by a branch of XII and a combined branch from C2 and C3.

26 The thyroid gland
- A Always contains just two lobes and an isthmus
- B Moves on swallowing due to its attachment to the suprahyoid muscles
- C Receives a vascular supply from both the external carotid and subclavian arteries
- D Drains to both the internal jugular and brachiocephalic veins
- E Contains a fixed number of parathyroid glands

27 The larynx contains
- A Four sets of paired cartilages
- B A membrane which forms both the aryepiglottic and vestibular folds
- C A ventricle lying between the vocal fold superiorly and the vestibular fold inferiorly
- D An inlet widened by the thyroepiglottic muscle
- E Intrinsic muscles which are innervated by X

26 A False
  B False
  C True
  D True
  E False

The pyramidal lobe, an embryological remnant derived from the thyroglossal duct, may be present. The thyroid gland moves on swallowing, due to its attachment to the pretracheal fascia. Its rich vascular supply is derived from the superior and inferior thyroid arteries, branches of the external carotid and thyrocervical trunk of the subclavian, respectively. The superior and middle thyroid veins drain directly (or indirectly) to the external jugular vein, whereas the inferior thyroid vein drains to the brachiocephalic. The number of parathyroid glands is variable, with from 3 to 6 glands present.

27 A False
  B True
  C False
  D True
  E True

The larynx contains three paired (arytenoid, corniculate and cuneiform) and unpaired (epiglottic, thyroid and cricoid) cartilages. The quadrangular membrane forms the vestibular fold with its lower border, and the aryepiglottic fold with its upper one. The ventricle of the larynx lies between the vestibule and the infraglottic cavity. It has the vestibular fold directly above it and the vocal fold below. The thyroepiglottic muscle is attached to both the laminae of the thyroid cartilage and the epiglottis, and serves to widen the largyngeal inlet. All the intrinsic laryngeal muscles except cricothyroid are supplied by the recurrent largyngeal nerve, whereas cricothyroid is supplied by the external laryngeal nerve. Both these nerves are branches of X.

28 Regarding the external pharyngeal muscles
   A   The fibres of superior constrictor lie superficial to the other constrictor muscles
   B   Middle constrictor is attached to bone
   C   Middle constrictor contains fibres preventing the entry of air into the oesophagus
   D   Inferior constrictor is attached to the laryngeal cartilages
   E   At least one nerve passes between superior and middle constrictor

29 The internal pharyngeal muscles
   A   Consist of five pairs of muscles
   B   Run circularly around the pharynx
   C   Include a muscle which opens the pharyngotympanic tube
   D   Insert into a midline fibrous raphe
   E   Are innervated by the pharyngeal plexus

28 A False
    B True
    C False
    D True
    E True
Superior constrictor lies innermost of the three external pharyngeal muscles. Middle constrictor arises partly from the hyoid bone. Fibres of inferior constrictor form cricopharyngeus, which controls the entry of air into the oesophagus. Inferior constrictor is attached to the thyroid and cricoid cartilages. IX, the lingual nerve and stylopharyngeus pass between the superior and middle constrictors.

29 A True
    B False
    C True
    D False
    E False
The five pairs of internal pharyngeal muscles do not have a circular course and, unlike their external counterparts, do not insert into a midline raphe. Tensor veli palatini is innervated by the nerve to medial pterygoid (a branch of V_3), whereas the remaining muscles are supplied by the pharyngeal plexus. The origin of tensor veli palatini includes the Eustachian tube and hence serves to open this tube.

3 Vascular anatomy

1 Which of the following statements is/are correct?

A The common carotid bifurcates level with the superior border of the cricoid cartilage

B The bifurcation in A lies at T1

C The external carotid is larger than the internal carotid

D The internal and common carotids do not form branches in the neck

E The thyroid ima arises from the aorta or the brachiocephalic artery

2 The external carotid artery

A Supplies the angular artery which passes towards the medial canthus

B Has a terminal branch which sends branches through both the foramina ovale and spinosum

C Does not anastomose with branches of the internal carotid

D Lies lateral to the internal carotid at their bifurcation

E Lies deep to the facial nerve in the parotid gland

Vascular anatomy: answers

1 A False
  B False
  C False
  D True
  E True

The common carotid bifurcates into two equally sized branches at the level of the superior border of the thyroid cartilage (C3–C4). Neither the internal nor the common carotids form branches in the neck, and the thyroid ima may arise from either the aorta or the brachiocephalic arteries.

2 A True
  B True
  C False
  D False
  E True

The angular artery, the part of the facial artery beyond its most distal branch, passes towards the medial canthus. The maxillary artery is one of the two terminal branches of the external carotid. Its middle meningeal and accessory meningeal branches cross the foramen spinosum and ovale, respectively. Numerous anastomoses exist between the branches of the internal and external carotids (e.g. the supraorbital and supratrochlear arteries with the superficial temporal). The external carotid lies medial to the internal carotid at the bifurcation of the common carotid. Within the parotid gland, VII lies superficial to the retromandibular vein, which in turn lies above the external carotid artery.

3 **The branches of the internal carotid artery include**
    A The posterior cerebral artery
    B The posterior communicating artery
    C An artery supplying the choroid plexus
    D A supply to the internal capsule
    E Vessels supplying the pituitary

4 **The vertebral artery**
    A Arises from the subclavian artery beneath scalenus anterior
    B Passes through the transverse foramen of C7
    C Enters the skull through the jugular foramen
    D Unites with its fellow artery at the upper border of the pons
    E Supplies intra- and extracranial structures

3 A False
  B True
  C True
  D True
  E True

The main branches of the internal carotid are the anterior cerebral, middle cerebral, anterior choroidal, posterior communicating and ophthalmic arteries. The anterior choroidal artery supplies the choroid plexus. The striate arteries, branches of the middle cerebral, supply the internal capsule and basal ganglia. The superior and inferior hypophyseal arteries are small branches of the internal carotid.

4 A False
  B False
  C False
  D False
  E True

The vertebral artery arises from the first part of the subclavian (i.e. before passing under scalenus anterior). It passes through the transverse foramina of the upper six cervical vertebra and the foramen magnum to unite with its fellow artery at the lower border of the pons and form the basilar artery. Its branches include the anterior and posterior spinal arteries (which supply the spinal cord), as well as the posterior inferior cerebellar artery.

5 **The following arteries are derived from the part of the subclavian described below**

   A   Lateral to scalenus anterior – vertebral

   B   Under scalenus anterior – deep intercostal

   C   Under scalenus anterior – superior cervical

   D   Medial to scalenus anterior – dorsal scapular

   E   Medial to scalenus anterior – suprascapular

6 **The lacrimal artery supplies the following**

   A   Skin of both eyelids

   B   Lateral rectus

   C   Inferior oblique

   D   Conjunctiva

   E   Meninges

5 A False
  B False
  C False
  D False
  E True

The subclavian artery is divided into three parts by scalenus anterior. The first part, lying medial to the muscle, forms the vertebral and internal thoracic arteries as well as the thyrocervical trunk. The latter divides into the transverse cervical, suprascapular and inferior thyroid arteries. The second part, lying under the muscle, forms the costocervical trunk from which the superior intercostal and deep cervical arteries are derived. The third part of the subclavian, lying lateral to scalenus anterior, rarely forms any branches.

6 A True
  B True
  C False
  D True
  E True

The lacrimal artery forms the lateral palpebral arteries which supply the skin of both eyelids as well as the palpebral, forniceal and some bulbar conjunctiva. The remaining conjunctiva is supplied by the anterior conjunctival arteries, branches of the anterior ciliary arteries. The lacrimal artery also supplies lateral rectus and the lacrimal gland as well as some of the meninges via a recurrent meningeal branch, which anastomoses with the middle meningeal artery. Inferior oblique is supplied by muscular branches of the ophthalmic and the infraorbital arteries.

7 **Which of the following statements is/are correct?**
   A The anterior ethmoidal artery is bathed in cerebrospinal fluid during its course
   B The posterior ethmoidal artery is the main arterial supply to the sinuses of the same name
   C The skin of the eyelids is only supplied by indirect branches of the ophthalmic artery
   D Branches of the ophthalmic artery supply the scalp
   E Branches of the external carotid artery supply some of the extraocular muscles

8 **Which of the following statements is/are correct?**
   A The anterior communicating artery crosses the interpeduncular cistern
   B The circle of Willis encircles the optic chiasm and the pituitary stalk
   C The anterior cerebral artery supplies the medial, lateral and inferior hemispheric surfaces
   D The middle cerebral artery runs deep within the central sulcus to supply the pre- and post-central gyri
   E The anterior cerebral and anterior choroidal arteries are the terminal branches of the internal carotid

7 A True
   B True
   C False
   D True
   E True

The anterior ethmoidal artery traverses the anterior ethmoidal canal to reach the anterior cranial fossa where it is bathed in cerebrospinal fluid. It then crosses the cribriform plate of the ethmoid to enter the nose. The posterior ethmoidal artery is the main vascular supply of the posterior ethmoidal and sphenoidal sinuses. The skin of the eyelids is supplied by the medial and lateral palpebral arteries, direct and indirect branches, respectively, of the ophthalmic artery. The supraorbital and supratrochlear arteries supply part of the scalp, whereas the infraorbital artery, the terminal portion of the maxillary, supplies inferior rectus and inferior oblique.

8 A False
   B True
   C True
   D False
   E False

The anterior communicating artery crosses the chiasmatic cistern to connect the two anterior cerebral arteries. The circle of Willis lies in the interpeduncular cistern, encircling the chiasm and pituitary. Up to 60% of individuals display some anomaly in the circle of Willis' structure. The anterior cerebral artery, one of the two terminal branches of the internal carotid, supplies the orbital surface of the frontal lobe as well as parts of the medial and lateral hemispheric surfaces. The other terminal branch of the internal carotid artery, the middle cerebral artery, runs deep in the lateral sulcus.

9   The anterior cerebral artery
   A   Is joined to its fellow artery by a 1.5 cm long vessel
   B   Passes below the optic nerve
   C   Runs in the interpeduncular cistern
   D   Passes adjacent to the corpus callosum
   E   Arises from the internal carotid artery after the ophthalmic artery is formed

10   The blood–brain barrier is absent at the following sites
   A   Area postrema of the fourth ventricle
   B   Anterior pituitary
   C   Caudate nucleus
   D   Pineal body
   E   Subthalamus

11   The following vessels supply or drain the cerebellum directly
   A   Vertebral artery
   B   Basilar artery
   C   Anterior inferior cerebellar artery
   D   Inferior sagittal sinus
   E   Great cerebral vein of Galen

9 A False
  B False
  C True
  D True
  E True

The anterior cerebral arteries are joined by the anterior communicating artery which is 4 mm long. They lie above the level of the optic nerve, passing through the interpeduncular and chiasmatic cisterns, before curving around the genu of the corpus callosum. The ophthalmic artery is one of the earlier branches of the internal carotid and the anterior and middle cerebral are its terminal branches. Therefore the anterior cerebral artery must arise after the ophthalmic artery is formed.

10 A True
  B False
  C False
  D True
  E False

The term 'the blood–brain barrier' arose after it was demonstrated that certain substances in the circulation had restricted access to the brain. Areas where this barrier appears to be missing include the posterior pituitary, pineal gland, median eminence of the hypothalamus and the area postrema of the fourth ventricle.

11 A False
  B False
  C True
  D False
  E False

The cerebellum is supplied by the following arteries:
Posterior inferior cerebellar – branch of vertebral artery
Anterior inferior cerebellar – branch of basilar artery
Superior cerebellar   – branch of basilar artery
The cerebellum drains to the superior and inferior cerebellar veins, which subsequently drain to the following: straight, sigmoid, inferior petrosal and occipital sinuses and the great cerebral vein (of Galen).

12 Which of the following statements is/are correct?
A The cerebral veins have a similar pattern of distribution to the cerebral arteries
B The cerebral veins are valved
C When draining into adjacent sinuses, the cerebral veins generally enter them obliquely
D The diploic veins communicate with the dural venous sinuses
E The sinuses also communicate with the vertebral venous plexuses

13 The following are unpaired venous sinuses
A Straight
B Transverse
C Occipital
D Petrosal
E Basilar

12 A False
B False
C True
D True
E True

The cerebral veins are valveless, running superficially in the arachnoid, generally entering the adjacent venous sinuses obliquely. Their pattern of distribution does not resemble the cerebral arterial supply. The diploic veins are large venous channels in the vault bones which communicate with the venous sinuses across the inner table of the skull. The internal vertebral venous plexuses communicate with the occipital and sigmoid sinuses.

13 A True
B False
C True
D False
E True

The straight sinus runs in the lower border of the falx cerebri along its insertion into the tentorium cerebelli. The transverse sinuses run laterally from the internal occipital protuberance, becoming the sigmoid sinuses once they leave the tentorium cerebelli. The occipital sinuses lie on either side of the foramen magnum, while the unpaired basilar plexus lies on the clivus. The superior petrosal sinuses run along the upper edge of the petrous temporal bones in the attachment of the tentorium cerebelli and drain into the transverse sinuses. The inferior petrosal sinuses run along the base of the petrous temporal bones and drain into the superior bulb of the internal jugular veins.

14 The cavernous sinus

   A   Anteriorly, lies at the superior orbital fissure

   B   Communicates with its contralateral sinus

   C   Drains mainly into the inferior petrosal sinuses

   D   Transmits VI which passes medial to the internal carotid artery

   E   May be thrombosed by sepsis from the inner ear

15 Blood from the following structures drains into the cavernous sinus

   A   Vault bones

   B   Skin covering the maxilla

   C   Infraorbital vein

   D   Deep middle cerebral vein

   E   Sphenoparietal sinus

14 A True
   B True
   C False
   D False
   E True

The cavernous sinus extends from the superior orbital fissure to the petrous temporal bone and communicates with its fellow via the intercavernous sinuses. It drains into the superior and inferior petrosal sinuses and pterygoid venous plexus. The abducens nerve initially lies lateral and later inferolateral to the internal carotid artery. Sepsis from the ear may spread via labyrinthine veins and the inferior petrosal sinus to the cavernous sinus.

15 A True
   B True
   C False
   D False
   E True

The following drain into the cavernous sinus:

Superior ophthalmic vein
Inferior ophthalmic vein
Sphenoparietal sinus (drains the skull vault)
Superior middle cerebral veins (drain the cortex along the lateral sulcus)

Blood from the skin overlying the maxilla drains naturally into the cavernous sinus by several different routes:

Angular vein to superior ophthalmic to cavernous sinus
Facial vein to pterygopalatine plexus to cavernous sinus

16 Regarding the cavernous sinus

   A   The internal carotid artery runs in its walls

   B   III passes medial to V_1

   C   VI lies medial to III

   D   Sympathetic fibres to the extraocular muscle paralysed in Horner's syndrome do not cross this sinus

   E   Blood from this sinus drains directly to the torcula herophili (confluence of sinuses)

17 Which of the statements about the following veins is/are correct?

   A   The external jugular vein is derived from both the posterior auricular and retromandibular veins

   B   The external jugular vein drains into the brachiocephalic vein

   C   The subclavian vein becomes the axillary vein after passing under the lateral border of the 1st rib

   D   The facial vein drains into the external jugular

   E   The anterior jugular vein is formed underneath the chin

16 A False
   B True
   C True
   D False
   E False

III, IV, V_1 and V_2 run in the lateral wall of the cavernous sinus, whereas VI and the internal carotid artery run through the sinus itself. III lies medial to V_1 and VI lies medial to both. The superior tarsal muscle (the unstriated part of levator palpebrae superioris) is innervated by sympathetic fibres, conveyed to the orbit by a plexus around the internal carotid artery, which passes these fibres in turn to III. The cavernous sinus drains to the petrosal sinuses and the pterygoid venous plexuses.

17 A True
   B False
   C False
   D False
   E True

The external jugular vein, formed by the union of the posterior division of the retromandibular vein and the posterior auricular vein, drains into the subclavian vein. The subclavian vessels pass over the first rib, becoming the axillary vessels at the rib's lateral border. The facial vein forms from the supraorbital and supratrochlear veins and drains into the internal jugular. The anterior jugular veins are formed from a collection of veins lying near the apex of the anterior triangle.

18 Kiesselbach's plexus receives branches from the following arteries
    A   Greater palatine
    B   Lesser palatine
    C   Sphenopalatine
    D   Nasopalatine
    E   Anterior ethmoidal

18 A True
   B False
   C True
   D False
   E False
   Kiesselbach's plexus lies on the lower part of the nasal septum at a point called Little's area. It is formed by the ascending branch of the greater palatine artery, the sphenopalatine artery and the septal branch of the superior labial artery. It is a common site of haemorhage and this may be controlled by applying pressure over the septum.

4 Neuroanatomy

1 In the cerebral hemispheres
  A Broca's area lies on the right inferior frontal gyrus
  B The motor cortex lies on the medial and lateral hemispheric surfaces
  C The sensory cortex lies anterior to the fissure of Rolando (central sulcus)
  D The insula is surrounded by the angular gyrus
  E The cuneus is separated from the precuneus by the parieto-occipital sulcus

2 The location of various areas of the cerebrum are as follows
  A Frontal eye field – anterior to the premotor strip
  B Auditory cortex – inferior frontal gyrus
  C Taste – frontoparietal operculum
  D Olfactory area – parietal lobe
  E Wernicke's area – frontal lobe

Neuroanatomy: answers

1 A False
    B True
    C False
    D False
    E True
Broca's area lies on the left inferior frontal gyrus and damage to it results in motor aphasia. The motor and sensory cortex lie on the pre- and post-central gyri, respectively. The motor cortex reaches the paracentral lobule on the medial hemispheric surface. The insula is surrounded by the circular sulcus and is covered by overlying opercula. The cuneus lies between the posterior part of the calcarine sulcus and the parieto-occipital sulcus, with the latter separating it from the precuneus.

2 A True
    B False
    C True
    D False
    E False
The cortical representation of these areas is as follows:

Frontal eye field – middle frontal gyrus, anterior to premotor strip
Auditory cortex – floor of lateral sulcus and adjacent superior temporal gyrus
Taste area – frontoparietal operculum
Olfactory area – piriform cortex
Wernicke's area – superior and middle temporal gyri
Broca's area – left inferior frontal gyrus

3 Which of these structures lie or pass adjacent to the cerebral peduncles?
  A   IV
  B   Colliculi
  C   Mamillary bodies
  D   Pineal gland
  E   Posterior perforated substance

4 The following fibres pass through the specified parts of the right internal capsule
  A   Anterior limb   – auditory radiation fibres
  B   Genu   – corticospinal fibres
  C   Posterior limb   – fibres from Broca's area
  D   Sublentiform part   – fibres from medial geniculate nucleus
  E   Retrolentiform part   – fibres passing to Brodmann's areas 15, 16
                            and 17

3 A True
  B False
  C True
  D False
  E True
The posterior perforated substance lies between the cerebral peduncles with the mamillary bodies lying slightly further anteriorly. The pineal gland and the four colliculi lie on the dorsal surface of the brainstem, well away from the cerebral peduncles. IV, although emerging from the dorsal surface of the brainstem, curves around the peduncles to pass towards the cavernous sinus.

4 A False
  B False
  C False
  D True
  E False
The internal capsule consists of an anterior limb, a genu and a posterior limb, as well as sublentiform and retrolentiform parts. The anterior limb contains frontopontine fibres and possibly fibres from the frontal eye field passing to the oculomotor nucleus. The genu contains fibres connecting the cerebral cortex with cranial nerve nuclei, while the posterior limb conveys both corticospinal and thalamocortical fibres. Fibres from Broca's area traverse the left internal capsule and thus aphasia frequently accompanies a right hemiplegia. The sublentiform part contains auditory radiation fibres passing from the medial geniculate nucleus to the auditory area. The retrolentiform part contains fibres passing from the lateral geniculate body to the primary visual area (Brodmann's area 17).

5 The midbrain

A   Crosses the tentorium at the level of the olive
B   On cross-section contains a pigmented band
C   Contains the red nucleus
D   Has its tegmentum lying dorsal to the aqueduct
E   Contains the nuclei of both III and IV

6 Which of the following tracts pass through the midbrain?

A   Medial lemniscus
B   Lateral lemniscus
C   Trigeminal lemniscus
D   Spinal lemniscus
E   Medial longitudinal fasciculus

5   A   False
    B   True
    C   True
    D   False
    E   True

The olive lies in the medulla, well below the level of the tentorium cerebelli. The midbrain extends from the mamillary bodies to the pons and contains the substantia nigra, which is visible on cross-section. It contains the oculomotor and trochlear nuclei (at the levels of the superior and inferior colliculi) as well as the red nucleus. The midbrain consists of three main parts: the tectum (roof) dorsal to the aqueduct with the tegmentum and crura cerebri ventral to it.

6   A   True
    B   True
    C   True
    D   True
    E   True

All these tracts pass through the midbrain. The medial lemniscus conveys light touch and proprioceptive information. The lateral lemniscus conveys auditory information from the cochlear and superior olivary nuclei to the inferior colliculus. The trigeminal lemniscus carries fibres from the spinal nucleus of V to the thalamus. The spinal lemniscus carries fibres from the spinothalamic and spinotectal tracts. The medial longitudinal fasciculus connects III, IV, VI and VIII. It co-ordinates eye movements and internuclear ophthalmoplegia may result when it is damaged.

7 The medulla contains

  A Cell bodies of third-order neurons involved in light touch and joint position sense

  B The vomiting centre

  C The olivary nuclei

  D Corticobulbar fibres decussating in the pyramids

  E Structures supplied by the posterior spinal artery

8 The pons

  A Grooves the basiocciput below the jugular tubercle

  B Has an artery running along the centre of its dorsal midline groove

  C Lies superior to the mamillary bodies

  D Lies inferior to the corpora quadrigemina

  E Is attached to just one cranial nerve by a single root

7 A False
  B True
  C True
  D False
  E False

The medulla contains cell bodies of second-order neurons lying in the gracile and cuneate nuclei. These fibres decussate in the upper medulla, ascend in the medial lemniscus and relay in the thalamus with third-order neurons projecting to the cortex. The area postrema (or vomiting centre) lies medial to the gracile nuclei and the olivary nuclei also lie in the medulla. Approximately 85% of corticospinal fibres decussate in the pyramid; corticobulbar fibres, by definition, terminate on cranial nerve nuclei. The posterior spinal artery arises at the level of the foramen magnum, descending through it to supply the spinal cord.

8 A False
  B False
  C False
  D True
  E False

The jugular tubercle lies close to the skull base and thus the pons, which grooves the basiocciput, lies above it. The pons lies between the midbrain (containing the four colliculi or corpora quadrigemina) and the medulla below. The basilar artery usually runs to one side of the pons's ventral midline groove. The trigeminal nerve, the only cranial nerve to be attached to the pons, has both a motor and a sensory root.

9   The following constitute the basal ganglia
- A   Red nucleus
- B   Caudate nucleus
- C   Thalamus
- D   Claustrum
- E   Amygdaloid body

10   In the cerebellum the
- A   Vallecula contains the superior and inferior vermis
- B   Folia are ridges on the cerebellar surface
- C   Superior and inferior lobes are separated by the primary fissure
- D   Superior cerebellar peduncle unites the pons
- E   Roof nuclei lie adjacent to the olivary nucleus

11   The Purkinje cells have
- A   Dendrites branching in the molecular layer
- B   A direct supply from mossy fibres
- C   Axons synapsing with the roof nuclei
- D   An indirect supply from climbing fibres
- E   Unmyelinated axons

9 A False
   B True
   C False
   D True
   E True

The basal ganglia are a group of nuclei in the forebrain and include the caudate and lentiform nuclei, the amygdaloid and claustrum.

10 A False
   B False
   C False
   D False
   E False

The vallecula is a cleft, separating the inferior parts of cerebellar hemispheres, into which the inferior vermis projects. Folia are grooves on the cerebellar surface equivalent to cerebral sulci. The primary fissure separates the anterior and posterior lobes, while the middle cerebellar peduncle connects with the pons. The so-called roof nuclei (emboliform, globose and fastigial) lie adjacent to the dentate nucleus; the olivary nucleus lies in the medulla.

11 A True
   B False
   C True
   D False
   E False

Purkinje cells have profuse dendritic branches and their myelinated axons synapse with the dentate and roof nuclei. Mossy fibres directly supply granule cells, whereas climbing fibres supply Purkinje cells.

12 The tentorium cerebelli
- A Consists of a single layer of dura
- B Lies in contact with five venous sinuses
- C Is suspended from the falx cerebri
- D Has a fixed edge attached to the anterior clinoid processes
- E Has a free edge lying superomedial to the trochlear nerve

13 Which of these vessels supply the dura?
- A Middle meningeal artery
- B Posterior ethmoidal artery
- C Ophthalmic artery
- D Lacrimal artery
- E Vertebral arteries

12 A False
 B True
 C True
 D False
 E True

The tentorium cerebelli consists of a fold of dura to which the falx cerebri and cerebelli attach. It forms the roof of the posterior cranial fossa and is in close contact with the straight sinus, and the paired transverse and superior petrosal sinuses. The trochlear nerve passes inferolateral to its free border to enter the lateral wall of the cavernous sinus. The free border is attached to the anterior clinoid processes, whereas the fixed border is attached to the posterior clinoids.

13 A True
 B False
 C True
 D True
 E True

Most of the supratentorial dura is supplied by the middle meningeal artery. Contributions are also received in the anterior cranial fossa from the anterior ethmoidal artery and meningeal branches of the ophthalmic (including the lacrimal). The middle cranial fossa receives an additional supply from the accessory meningeal artery and meningeal branches of the internal carotid. The dura of the posterior cranial fossa is supplied by meningeal branches of the vertebral arteries.

14 Which of these nerves innervate the dura?
- A V_1
- B V_2
- C   IX, X and XI
- D   Upper three cervical nerves
- E   Nervus spinosus

15 Regarding the sella turcica and its contents
- A   The lesser wing of the sphenoid forms the anterior clinoid processes
- B   The optic chiasm lies in the sulcus chiasmaticus
- C   The jugum of the sphenoid articulates with the cribriform plate of the ethmoid
- D   Initial enlargement of pituitary lesions generally causes an inferotemporal field defect
- E   One would expect enlarging pituitary lesions to compress the chiasm before the optic tracts

14 A True
   B True
   C False
   D True
   E True

Most of the supratentorial dura is supplied by V_1. In addition, a supplementary supply comes from:

Anterior cranial fossa – anterior ethmoidal and maxillary nerves
Middle cranial fossa – middle meningeal nerve (V_2) and nervus spinosus (V_3)
Posterior cranial fossa – meningeal branches of IX, X and C_1–C_3

15 A True
   B False
   C True
   D False
   E True

The anterior part of the body of the sphenoid (the jugum) articulates with the cribriform plate of the ethmoid. The anterior clinoid processes are formed from the sphenoid's lesser wing, while the middle and posterior clinoids are derived from its body. In 80% of cases the chiasm lies above the chiasmatic sulcus. Therefore, enlarging pituitary lesions first compress decussating inferonasal fibres, causing a superotemporal field defect. Only if the chiasm is prefixed (less than 10% of cases) can optic tract compression precede chiasmal involvement.

16 The lateral ventricles
  A Consist of a body and two horns
  B Are minor sites of cerebrospinal fluid production
  C Contain choroid plexus continuous with that of the third ventricle
  D Have a lumen indented by the calcarine sulcus
  E Possess a posterior horn that may be absent

17 The third ventricle
  A Is bounded anteriorly by the lamina terminalis
  B Extends above the pineal gland and the optic chiasm
  C May be crossed by fibres linking the thalami
  D Communicates with the lateral ventricles via the foramina of Luschka
  E Is bounded superiorly by the corpus callosum

18 The fourth ventricle
  A Lies in the medulla and pons
  B Has a sheet of grey matter lying on its roof
  C Does not contain choroid plexus
  D Transmits about 40 ml of cerebrospinal fluid per day
  E Allows cerebrospinal fluid to enter the subarachnoid space through three foramina

16 A False
   B False
   C True
   D True
   E True

The lateral ventricles consist of a body and three horns (anterior, posterior and inferior). The posterior horn is variably developed and may be absent. The lumen of the lateral ventricle is indented by the calcarine, collateral and parahippocampal sulci. Cerebrospinal fluid is produced by choroid plexuses of the lateral, third and fourth ventricles, with the former being responsible for the bulk of production.

17 A True
   B True
   C True
   D False
   E False

The third ventricle is a narrow slit-like cavity bounded anteriorly by the lamina terminalis and superiorly by ependyma. It extends above the optic chiasm and pineal gland, forming the supraoptic and pineal recesses. It drains cerebrospinal fluid from the two lateral ventricles via the foramina of Monro and an interthalamic adhesion is found in $\approx 60\%$ of individuals.

18 A True
   B False
   C False
   D False
   E True

The fourth ventricle lies within the pons and medulla and has its roof covered by the superior medullary velum, a thin sheet of white matter. It contains a small amount of choroid plexus and transmits over 500 ml of cerebrospinal fluid per day which drains from the midline foramen of Magendie and the lateral foramina of Luschka.

19 The following structures pass through the named orifices

A	Nasopalatine nerve	– Greater palatine canal
B	Vidian nerve	– Pterygoid canal
C	Branches of the pterygopalatine ganglion	– Sphenopalatine foramen
D	Branches of the pterygopalatine ganglion	– Pterygomaxillary fissure
E	Maxillary nerve	– Infraorbital foramen

20 The following are innervated by fibres conveyed in V_3

   A   Anterior two-thirds of the tongue
   B   Roof of the mouth
   C   Submandibular gland
   D   Parotid gland
   E   Tensor veli palatini

19 A False
   B True
   C True
   D False
   E False

The nasopalatine nerve, a branch of the pterygopalatine ganglion, passes through the sphenopalatine foramen. The Vidian nerve (nerve of the pterygoid canal) crosses this canal. The pterygomaxillary fissure connects the pterygopalatine and infratemporal fossae and is not crossed by any structures. The maxillary nerve becomes the infraorbital nerve after entering the orbit through the inferior orbital fissure and it is this nerve that crosses the infraorbital foramen.

20 A True
   B False
   C True
   D True
   E True

V_3 supplies: the anterior two-thirds of the tongue (lingual nerve – sensation, chorda tympani fibres – taste), the submandibular gland (via chorda tympani fibres carried by the lingual nerve), the parotid gland (auriculotemporal nerve) and tensor veli palatini (nerve to medial pterygoid). The palate is supplied by the greater and lesser palatine nerves (branches of V_2).

21 Failure of the ipsilateral pupil to constrict to bright light could be due to damage

A   To the superior colliculus
B   Along the course of the posterior communicating artery
C   To the pretectal nuclei
D   To the lateral geniculate nucleus
E   To the ipsilateral Edinger–Westphal nucleus

21 A False
   B True
   C True
   D False
   E True

Most afferent information from the retina passes via the optic nerve, chiasm and tract to the lateral geniculate body. A group of fibres involved in pupillary reflexes leaves the optic tract forming the superior brachium. These fibres pass to the pretectal nuclei which lie adjacent to the superior colliculi. There they synapse with both Edinger–Westphal nuclei. The impulses pass ipsilaterally to each oculomotor nerve, onto the ciliary ganglion and finally via the short ciliary nerves reach sphincter pupillae. Damage to either the superior colliculus or lateral geniculate body will spare this pathway. Damage along the course of the posterior communicating artery, which passes adjacent to III, or to the pretectal nuclei or ipsilateral Edinger–Westphal nucleus, will interrupt the direct light reflex.

5 Orbital and autonomic anatomy

1 The sympathetic nervous system
- A Has an outflow extending from C4 to L2
- B Leaves the spinal cord in posterior nerve roots
- C Always relays in the paravertebral ganglia
- D Has preganglionic neuron cell bodies in the lateral horn
- E Contains afferent and efferent fibres

2 All the cervical ganglia
- A Are entirely sympathetic
- B Form by fusion of two ganglia
- C Innervate the heart
- D Form cranial nerve branches
- E Have grey rami communicantes proximal to their white rami

Orbital and autonomic anatomy: answers

1   A False
    B False
    C False
    D True
    E True
    The sympathetic nervous system has a thoracolumbar outflow (T_1–L_2) and its preganglionic neurons' cell bodies lie in the lateral horn of the grey matter. These neurons leave the cord via ventral (anterior) roots and may pass through the paravertebral ganglia without synapsing. Both afferent and efferent fibres are present in the sympathetic nervous system.

2   A True
    B False
    C True
    D False
    E False
    The three cervical ganglia are purely sympathetic and form from the fusion of eight ganglia (four forming the superior ganglion and two each the middle and inferior ganglia). All three ganglia have visceral branches supplying the cardiac plexus. Only the superior ganglion supplies cranial nerves, whereas the remaining two ganglia supply cervical nerves.

3   **The superior cervical ganglion**
  A   Lies level with the superior border of the thyroid cartilage
  B   Supplies orbital structures
  C   Supplies branches to IX, X and XI
  D   Supplies fibres that run in the deep petrosal nerve
  E   Innervates the heart

4   **The middle cervical ganglion**
  A   Is the smallest of the sympathetic cervical ganglia
  B   Lies level with the cricoid cartilage
  C   Gives white rami communicantes to C5 and C6
  D   Sends branches along the superior thyroid artery
  E   Has a double connection to the inferior ganglion

5   **The right inferior cervical ganglion**
  A   Lies between the transverse process of C8 and the neck of the first rib
  B   Is fused with the first thoracic ganglion in 20% of individuals
  C   Is connected to the ansa subclavia
  D   Sends preganglionic fibres to the heart
  E   Sends branches along the vertebral artery

3   A   False
    B   True
    C   True
    D   True
    E   True
    The superior cervical ganglion lies just below the skull base supplying
    fibres to the orbit, IX, X and XII, as well as the cardiac plexus, via its
    superior cardiac branch. The deep petrosal nerve carries sympathetic
    fibres from the internal carotid artery plexus. With the greater
    petrosal nerve, it forms the nerve of the pterygoid canal.

4   A   True
    B   True
    C   False
    D   False
    E   True
    The small middle cervical ganglion lies level with the cricoid cartilage
    and gives grey rami communicantes to C5 and C6. It supplies the
    thyroid gland via fibres accompanying the inferior thyroid artery and
    is joined to the inferior ganglion by at least two connections.

5   A   False
    B   False
    C   True
    D   False
    E   True
    The inferior cervical ganglion lies between the transverse process of
    C7 and the neck of the first rib. In 80% of individuals it is fused with
    the T1 ganglion, forming the stellate ganglion. From this ganglion,
    grey rami communicantes pass to C7 and C8, and arterial branches
    pass along the subclavian and vertebral vessels. The inferior cervical
    ganglion, like its fellows, supplies the heart but only with
    postganglionic fibres. The ansa subclavia is one of two or more
    connections between the middle and inferior cervical ganglia.

6 **Horner's syndrome is an ocular sympathetic palsy. From knowledge of the sympathetic pathway it can be predicted that**

    A   A hypothalamic lesion would cause loss of sweating over the upper half of the body

    B   A brachial plexus avulsion would leave postganglionic fibres initially intact

    C   A tumour at the lung apex could only cause loss of sweating above the ipsilateral eye

    D   If only the sympathetic pathway is considered, complete transection of the internal carotid at its origin would cause loss of all sweating above the eye

    E   Complete transection of the external carotid would not affect sympathetic innervation of the head and neck

7 **All the cranial parasympathetic ganglia have**

    A   The nuclei of their preganglionic neurons lying in the floor of the fourth ventricle

    B   Three roots

    C   Roots derived from the trigeminal nerve

    D   A root whose fibres are conveyed along branches of the internal carotid artery during part of their course

    E   Afferent fibres passing through them without synapsing

6 A False
   B True
   C False
   D False
   E False
A hypothalamic lesion may affect the first neuron in the sympathetic pathway causing loss of sweating over one side (half) of the body. Avulsion of the brachial plexus would interrupt the sympathetic pathway, but the postganglionic fibres, originating from the superior cervical ganglion, would be unaffected. Fibres controlling sweating are carried on the wall of the external carotid artery, with a few individuals having these fibres conveyed by the internal carotid as well. Therefore an apical lung tumour would affect sweating over the head and neck. Transection of the external carotid would interrupt these (sympathetic) sweating fibres, while internal carotid transection would spare sweating in the majority of patients.

7 A False
   B False
   C True
   D False
   E True
The nuclei of the preganglionic neurons supplying the parasympathetic ganglia are the Edinger–Westphal nucleus of III (ciliary); lacrimatory nucleus of VII (pterygopalatine); superior salivatory nucleus of VII (submandibular) and inferior salivatory nucleus of IX (otic). Only the salivatory and lacrimatory nuclei lie in the floor of the fourth ventricle, whereas the nuclei of III lie at the level of the superior colliculus. Although the ganglia generally have three roots, the otic ganglion is an exception with an extra motor root from the nerve to medial pterygoid. The sensory root is derived from V (V_1 = ciliary, V_2 = pterygopalatine, V_3 = submandibular and otic) and its fibres pass through the ganglion without synapsing. All the sympathetic fibres pass at some point along the internal carotid artery or its branches (ciliary and pterygopalatine = internal carotid, submandibular = facial, otic = middle meningeal artery).

8 **The ciliary ganglion**
   A Lies between the optic nerve and medial rectus
   B Is situated 2.5 cm from the orbital apex
   C Receives postganglionic fibres from its two non-sensory roots
   D Conveys sensation from some anterior chamber structures to the nasociliary nerve
   E Forms long and short ciliary nerves

9 **The pterygopalatine ganglion supplies branches to the following structures**
   A Nasal mucosa
   B Glands of Krause and Wolfring
   C Eustachian tube
   D Lower lip
   E Ethmoidal air cells

8 A False
   B False
   C False
   D True
   E False

The ciliary ganglion lies between the optic nerve and lateral rectus, 1 cm from the optic foramen. Only the sympathetic root conveys postganglionic fibres (from the superior cervical ganglion). The parasympathetic root consists of preganglionic fibres which synapse in the ganglion. The sensory root, derived from the nasociliary nerve, conveys sensory information from the cornea and iris. Although the short ciliary nerves are branches of this ganglion, the long ciliary nerves are derived from the nasociliary nerve.

9 A True
   B False
   C False
   D False
   E True

The pterygopalatine ganglion forms orbital, palatine, nasal and pharyngeal branches. The former supplies the sphenoidal and ethmoidal sinuses. The nasal mucosa is supplied by the nasal branches (lateral and medial posterior superior nasal nerves) of which the nasopalatine nerve is the largest.

10 The pterygopalatine ganglion
   A   Is suspended from the maxillary nerve
   B   Receives preganglionic fibres from the deep petrosal nerve
   C   Is directly supplied with fibres from nervus intermedius by the greater petrosal nerve
   D   Supplies orbitalis with sympathetic fibres via the superior orbital fissure
   E   Provides the only parasympathetic supply to the lacrimal gland via the zygomatic branch of the maxillary nerve

11 The otic ganglion
   A   Lies below the foramen rotundum
   B   Is attached to the nerve of lateral pterygoid
   C   Receives fibres passing through the tympanic plexus
   D   Supplies the parotid with fibres derived from the inferior salivatory nucleus
   E   Receives sympathetic fibres conveyed by a branch of the maxillary artery

10 A True
   B False
   C False
   D False
   E False

The pterygopalatine ganglion is suspended from the maxillary nerve and receives parasympathetic fibres from the lacrimatory nucleus of VII, via the greater petrosal nerve. This nerve is joined by the deep petrosal to form the nerve of the pterygoid canal, which becomes the motor root of the ganglion. The ganglion's orbital branches cross the inferior orbital fissure to supply orbitalis. These branches form a retro-orbital plexus supplying orbital structures with both sympathetic and parasympathetic innervation. Rami lacrimales thus provide a parasympathetic supply to the lacrimal gland, additional to that supplied by the zygomatic nerve.

11 A False
   B False
   C True
   D True
   E True

The otic ganglion lies below the foramen ovale and is attached to the nerve to medial pterygoid. The ganglion receives parasympathetic fibres from the inferior salivatory nucleus of IX, via the tympanic plexus of the middle ear, and supplies the parotid gland via the auriculotemporal nerve. Its sympathetic fibres are derived from a plexus around the middle meningeal artery.

12 The most inferiorly located cranial parasympathetic ganglion

   A Lies on genioglossus

   B Is attached to the lingual nerve

   C Receives postganglionic fibres from the chorda tympani

   D Receives sympathetic fibres from a plexus along the lingual artery

   E Supplies both the submandibular and sublingual glands

13 Which of the following foramina are known to convey autonomic fibres?

   A Optic foramen

   B Foramen magnum

   C Stylomastoid foramen

   D Foramen rotundum

   E Foramen ovale

12 A False
   B True
   C False
   D False
   E True

The submandibular ganglion, lying adjacent to the side of the tongue, is suspended from the lingual nerve. It is supplied with preganglionic parasympathetic fibres by the chorda tympani, while its postganglionic sympathetic fibres (which originate from the superior cervical ganglion) are derived locally from a plexus around the facial artery. The sympathetic fibres traverse the ganglion without synapsing. It supplies parasympathetic fibres to both the submandibular and sublingual glands.

13 A True
   B True
   C False
   D False
   E True

Autonomic fibres pass through the foramina as detailed below:

Optic foramen   – sympathetic fibres to ciliary ganglion
Foramen magnum   – sympathetic plexus around vertebral
                           arteries
Stylomastoid foramen – parasympathetic fibres in VII from N. intermedius leave in chorda tympani 6 mm above this foramen
Foramen rotundum   – V_2 receives autonomic fibres from the pterygopalatine ganglion after crossing this foramen
Foramen ovale   – the lesser petrosal either passes through this foramen or the canaliculus innominatus

14 The following pass through a canal in the temporal bone
  A Fibres from the superior cervical ganglion
  B Labyrinthine artery
  C Fibres from the inferior salivatory nucleus
  D Pharyngotympanic tube
  E Vidian nerve

15 The following ganglia are closely related to the named structures below
  A Ciliary   – lateral rectus
  B Pterygopalatine – maxillary nerve
  C Submandibular – inferior alveolar nerve
  D Otic   – nerve to lateral pterygoid
  E Otic   – foramen ovale

14 A True
    B True
    C True
    D True
    E False

Fibres from the superior cervical ganglion form a plexus around the internal carotid artery and cross the carotid canal in the petrous temporal bone. The labyrinthine artery enters the internal acoustic meatus. Fibres from the inferior salivatory nucleus (the parasympathetic supply to the parotid gland) pass to the tympanic branch of IX, reaching the tympanic plexus via the inferior tympanic canaliculus in the temporal bone. The Eustachian tube lies in (temporal) bone for one-third of its length, connecting the tympanic cavity and nasopharynx. The Vidian nerve (nerve of the pterygoid canal) traverses the pterygoid process of the sphenoid bone.

15 A True
    B True
    C False
    D False
    E True

The locations of the cranial parasympathetic ganglia are:

Ciliary — between the optic nerve and lateral rectus
Pterygopalatine — suspended from V_2 by two ganglionic branches
Submandibular — suspended from the lingual nerve
Otic — lies below the foramen ovale attached to the nerve to medial pterygoid

16 The following cross the superior orbital fissure above the common tendinous ring

A   Superior ophthalmic vein
B   Frontal nerve
C   Nasociliary nerve
D   Upper division of III
E   Parasympathetic fibres to the lacrimal gland

17 The following structures frequently pass within the right common tendinous ring

A   Ophthalmic artery
B   Inferior ophthalmic vein
C   Fibres from both Edinger–Westphal nuclei
D   Fibres from the left main oculomotor nucleus
E   Fibres which after synapsing reach the nucleus interpolaris

16 A True
   B True
   C False
   D False
   E True
The following cross the superior orbital fissure above the common tendinous ring:
L – lacrimal nerve
(O)
F – frontal nerve
T – trochlear nerve
S – superior ophthalmic vein

17 A True
   B False
   C False
   D True
   E False
Through the common tendinous ring pass the upper and lower divisions of III, the abducent and nasociliary nerves (TAN), together with the optic nerve and ophthalmic artery traversing the optic canal. Fibres from the accessory oculomotor (Edinger–Westphal) nuclei supply parasympathetic fibres to ipsilateral orbital structures. The inferior ophthalmic vein traverses the inferior orbital fissure. Nucleus interpolaris forms part of the trigeminal spinal nucleus and receives spinothalamic input from the maxillary area via the maxillary nerve.

18 The relations of the following nerves in the orbit are

A   Trochlear   – passes forwards beneath superior rectus and levator palpebrae superioris to supply superior oblique

B   Ophthalmic – divides into the three nerves below, after passing through the superior orbital fissure

C   Lacrimal   – lies adjacent to medial rectus

D   Frontal   – passes between superior rectus and levator palpabrae superioris

E   Nasociliary – crosses beneath the optic nerve to run medial to medial rectus

19 The nasociliary nerve

A   Receives sensory information from the iris

B   Has fibres crossing part of the ethmoid bone

C   Supplies both the inner and outer surfaces of the nose

D   Sends a branch through the anterior cranial fossa

E   Innervates the sphenoid sinus

18 A False
   B False
   C False
   D False
   E False
The relations of the five nerves in the orbit are:
Trochlear   – runs above superior rectus and levator palpebrae superioris before supplying superior oblique on its upper surface
Ophthalmic – never enters the orbit, as it divides into the three branches below before reaching the superior orbital fissure
Lacrimal   – runs along the upper border of lateral rectus with the lacrimal artery
Frontal   – passes forwards on the upper border of levator palpebrae superioris
Nasociliary – initially passes forwards lateral to the optic nerve before crossing above the nerve with the ophthalmic artery

19 A True
   B True
   C True
   D True
   E True
The nasociliary nerve, which supplies sensory fibres to the iris, has an anterior ethmoidal branch reaching the nose via the anterior cranial fossa and cribriform plate of the ethmoid. The nasal branches of the anterior ethmoidal nerve (2 internal and 1 external nasal) supply part of the mucous membrane and dorsal surface of the nose. The posterior ethmoidal nerve, when present, supplies the posterior ethmoidal and sphenoidal air sinuses.

20 The short ciliary nerves

A Pierce the sclera around the optic nerve with the long ciliary nerves

B Run forward in the choroid to supply the cornea

C Convey sympathetic fibres to the pupil

D Convey parasympathetic fibres to the ciliary muscle

E Communicate with fibres reaching the nucleus caudalis

21 The long ciliary nerves supply the

A Ciliary body with motor fibres

B Iris

C Cornea

D Conjunctiva

E Sphincter pupillae

22 The inferior orbital fissure transmits the following

A A vein communicating with the pterygoid venous plexus

B Maxillary nerve

C Infraorbital artery

D Branches of the sphenopalatine ganglion

E Zygomatic nerve

20 A False
  B False
  C False
  D True
  E True

The short ciliary nerves pierce the sclera around the optic nerve along with the short ciliary arteries. They pass forward in the suprachoroidal space (between the choroid and sclera) and do not carry sympathetic fibres to dilator pupillae. These are carried by the long ciliary nerves. They do convey parasympathetic fibres to the iris and ciliary muscle. Nucleus caudalis is the lowest part of the spinal trigeminal nucleus, and sensory fibres from the area supplied by V_1 end there.

21 A False
  B True
  C True
  D True
  E False

The long ciliary nerves, branches of the nasociliary, supply sensory fibres to the ciliary body, conjunctiva, cornea and iris as well as postganglionic fibres to dilator pupillae.

22 A True
  B True
  C True
  D True
  E True

All the structures listed traverse this fissure. The vein communicating with the pterygoid venous plexus is the inferior ophthalmic vein. The sphenopalatine ganglion is an alternative term for the pterygopalatine ganglion.

23 The ophthalmic artery
  A   Is the first branch formed by the internal carotid
  B   Traverses the optic canal peripheral to the optic nerve dura
  C   Lies lateral to the optic nerve in the orbit before crossing below
       it in 15% of cases
  D   Has the external nasal and supratrocheal arteries as terminal
       branches
  E   Is the sole arterial supply to the orbital contents

24 Known variations in the ophthalmic artery include
  A   Arising from a branch of the maxillary artery
  B   Crossing either above or below the optic nerve
  C   Not supplying the lacrimal artery
  D   Entering the orbit via the inferior orbital fissure
  E   Receiving tributaries from the facial artery

23 A False
    B False
    C True
    D False
    E False

The ophthalmic artery is the first branch of the internal carotid after it leaves the cavernous sinus. During its course through the petrous temporal bone and the cavernous sinus, the internal carotid forms caroticotympanic, pterygoid, cavernous, meningeal and hypophyseal branches. The ophthalmic artery lies within dura as it traverses the optic canal, passing forwards between the optic nerve and lateral rectus, before crossing above the nerve in ≈85% of cases. Its two terminal branches are the supratrochlear and dorsal nasal vessels. The infraorbital artery supplies an appreciable number of orbital contents, including inferior rectus, inferior oblique and the lacrimal sac.

24 A True
    B True
    C True
    D False
    E False

The ophthalmic artery, like the lacrimal, may rarely arise from the middle meningeal artery. It is known to cross below the optic nerve in 15% of cases and may enter the orbit via the superior orbital fissure, instead of the optic canal. It has no connection with the facial artery.

25 The short posterior ciliary arteries
  A Form some seven branches
  B Form the major arterial circle of the iris
  C Form an arterial network around the papilla
  D Run in the suprachoroidal space
  E Supply anterior sclera

26 The anterior ciliary arteries
  A Arise in pairs from the four recti
  B Supply all the bulbar and forniceal conjunctiva
  C Supply both episclera and sclera
  D Anastomose with long posterior ciliary arteries
  E Are accompanied by anterior ciliary veins which drain the whole
      of the anterior segment

25 A False
   B False
   C True
   D True
   E False

The seven or so short posterior ciliary arteries divide into 10–20 vessels, whose branches form the circle of Haller–Zinn, an anastomotic circle around the optic nerve head. They pass forward in the suprachoroidal space between the sclera and choroid, supplying the latter and some of the sclera, as far forward as the equator. The major arterial circle of the iris is formed from the long ciliary and anterior ciliary arteries.

26 A False
   B False
   C True
   D True
   E False

The seven anterior ciliary arteries are formed from muscular branches of the ophthalmic artery conveyed by the four recti. Each muscle forms two of these arteries, except lateral rectus which forms just one. Their anterior conjunctival branches supply the bulbar conjunctiva within 4 mm of the limbus, the remainder being supplied by branches of the palpebral vessels. The anterior ciliary vessels supply the sclera anterior to the recti insertions as well as episclera. They anastomose with the long posterior ciliary arteries to form the major arterial circle of the iris. The anterior ciliary veins do accompany the anterior ciliary arteries but mainly drain blood from the ciliary muscle.

27 The superior ophthalmic vein
- A Forms directly from branches of the supraorbital and supratrochlear veins
- B Drains blood from the ethmoidal air cells
- C Communicates with the central retinal vein
- D Drains into the pterygoid venous plexus
- E Only drains the orbit

28 The inferior ophthalmic vein
- A Has a similar number of tributaries to the superior ophthalmic
- B Runs under inferior rectus
- C Drains blood from the lacrimal sac
- D Communicates with the facial vein
- E May drain directly into the cavernous sinus

27 A False
B True
C True
D False
E False

The angular vein forms from the union of the supraorbital and supratrochlear veins. The superior ophthalmic arising from the supraorbital and angular veins drains part of the forehead. Its tributaries include the ethmoidal and central retinal veins and it drains into the cavernous sinus.

28 A False
B False
C True
D True
E True

The inferior ophthalmic vein has fewer tributaries than the superior ophthalmic and these include the lacrimal vein. It forms from a plexus on the orbital floor and runs above inferior rectus to enter the cavernous sinus (either directly or indirectly via the superior ophthalmic vein). It communicates with the superior ophthalmic vein, the pterygoid venous plexus via the inferior orbital fissure, and the facial vein across the orbital margin. It also drains blood from the lacrimal sac.

6 Ocular adnexae and extraocular muscles

1 The lacrimal gland
    A   Is a compound tubular gland
    B   Continues draining if the palpebral portion is removed
    C   Is supplied by autonomic fibres from the nerve of the pterygoid canal
    D   Only contributes the middle layer of the tear film
    E   Lies below the lesser wing of the sphenoid

2 Regarding the lacrimal drainage apparatus
    A   The puncta are directed posteriorly
    B   The upper punctum lies directly above the lower
    C   The canaliculi initially run medially
    D   The canaliculi drain into a diverticulum
    E   The lacrimal sac lies in contact with the medial palpebral ligament

Ocular adnexae and extraocular muscles: answers

1   A   False
     B   False
     C   True
     D   True
     E   False

The lacrimal gland lies in a fossa on the orbital surface of the frontal bone. It is a tubulo-acinar gland consisting of a large orbital portion and a smaller palpebral portion. It drains via 10–12 ducts that traverse the palpebral portion to reach the superior fornix. Removing the palpebral portion abolishes drainage and hence production of most of the aqueous middle layer of the precorneal tear film. The gland is innervated by autonomic fibres reaching the pterygopalatine ganglion in the nerve of the pterygoid canal.

2   A   True
     B   False
     C   False
     D   True
     E   False

The lacrimal puncta point slightly posteriorly and lie adjacent to the junction of the ciliary and lacrimal portions of the lid margin. The upper puncta lie ≈ 0.5 mm medial to the lower. The lacrimal canaliculi run vertically for ≈ 2 mm and then pass horizontally where they often unite before entering the sinus of Maier, a diverticulum of the lacrimal sac. The lacrimal sac lies in the lacrimal fossa surrounded by lacrimal fascia, separating it from the medial palpebral ligament.

3 **Which of the following statements is/are correct?**
   A The lacrimal fossa is just formed by the lacrimal bone
   B Inferior oblique attaches to the orbital floor lateral to the infraorbital foramen
   C The angular vein passes 8 mm medial to the medial canthus
   D The nasolacrimal sac drains to the middle meatus
   E The nasolacrimal duct passes through two bones, to reach the nose

4 **Levator palpabrae superioris**
   A Is attached to the medial and lateral orbital walls
   B Only inserts into skin and superior tarsal plate
   C Is the antagonist of the orbital portion of orbicularis
   D Is innervated by the superior division of III which enters the orbit above the common tendinous ring
   E Is supplied by neurons whose cell bodies lie just below the level of the skull base

3 A False
   B False
   C True
   D False
   E False

The lacrimal fossa is formed by the frontal process of the maxilla anteriorly and the lacrimal bone posteriorly. The origin of inferior oblique on the orbital surface of the maxilla extends medially to the lacrimal fascia and the margin of the nasolacrimal canal. The angular vein, formed from the supraorbital and supratrochlear veins, crosses the medial palpebral ligament 8 mm medial to the medial canthus. The nasolacrimal duct runs through a canal formed by three bones (maxilla, lacrimal and inferior concha) before opening in the inferior meatus ≈ 2 cm behind the nostril.

4 A True
   B False
   C False
   D False
   E True

Levator palpebrae superioris (LPS) arises from the orbital surface of the lesser wing of the sphenoid, and the horns of its aponeurosis are attached to the adjacent orbital walls. It inserts into skin, superior tarsal plate and the superior conjunctival fornix. It opposes the action of the palpebral portion of orbicularis oculi, while frontalis antagonizes the orbital portion. LPS is innervated both by the upper division of III (passing through the common tendinous ring) and by sympathetic fibres. The cell bodies of these postganglionic sympathetic neurons lie in the superior cervical ganglion (formed from the fused ganglia of C1–C4) just below the level of the skull base.

5 Which of the following statements regarding the eyelids is/are correct?

A The muscle of Riolan lies adjacent to the lid margin

B Their main sensory nerves lies superficial to orbicularis oculi

C Mueller's muscle is only present in the upper lid

D The tarsal plates are made of cartilage

E The superior palpebral conjunctiva is firmly attached to the tarsus

6 The orbital septum is pierced by the following structures

A Supratrochlear nerve

B Infratrochlear nerve

C Lacrimal nerve

D Medial palpebral arteries

E Supraorbital vessels

5 A True
   B False
   C False
   D False
   E True
   The ciliary portion of orbicularis oculi (muscle of Riolan) consists of fine muscle fibres lying adjacent to the lid margin. The main sensory supply to the lids passes between orbicularis oculi and the underlying orbital septum. Several muscles are named after Muller including: the superior tarsal muscle, the inferior palpebral muscle connecting inferior rectus and the tarsal plate, and orbitalis which closes part of the inferior orbital fissure. The tarsal plates are composed of fibroelastic tissue and the superior palpebral conjunctiva is firmly adherent to the tarsal plate.

6 A True
   B True
   C True
   D True
   E True
   The orbital septum is attached to the orbital margin and is continuous with the tarsal plates. It is pierced by the

   Supratrochlear and supraorbital vessels and nerves
   Infratrochlear nerve
   Lacrimal vessels and nerves
   Medial palpebral arteries
   Aponeurosis of levator palpebrae superioris

7 The following structures lie anterior to the grey line

- A Glands of Wolfring
- B Glands of Moll
- C Meibomian glands
- D Crypts of Henle
- E Glands of Zeis

8 The skin of the eyelids is innervated by branches of the

- A Nasociliary nerve
- B Zygomatic nerve
- C Frontal nerve
- D Maxillary nerve
- E Mandibular nerve

7 A False
   B True
   C False
   D False
   E True
The grey line is an avascular area on the lid margin, between the lashes anteriorly and the orifices of the Meibomian glands posteriorly. The lid may easily be split at this point into anterior and posterior lamellae. The glands of Krause and Wolfring are accessory lacrimal glands lying in the forniceal conjunctiva and tarsal plates, respectively. The crypts of Henle and glands of Manz secrete mucin and lie in the tarsal and limbal conjunctiva, respectively. The glands of Zeis (modified sebaceous glands) open onto a lash follicle, while the glands of Moll (modified sweat glands) open onto lash follicles or the lid margin. Therefore, only the glands of Zeis and Moll lie anterior to the grey line.

8 A True
   B False
   C True
   D True
   E False
The skin of the lids is innervated by the following nerves:

Upper lid: (V_1) nasociliary – infratrochlear   Medially
                    frontal   – supraorbital
                                 – supratrochlear   to
                    lacrimal   laterally

Lower lid: (V_1) infratrochlear   Medially
           (V_2) infraorbital   Laterally

9   **Orbicularis oculi**
    A   Is crossed by fibres of levator palpabrae superioris
    B   Inserts into the medial and lateral palpebral ligaments
    C   Apposes the lower lid to the globe
    D   Contains a lacrimal portion that surrounds the lacrimal sac
    E   Has ciliary and palpebral portions which are separated by the glands of Moll

10 **Which of the following statements is/are correct?**
    A   Corrugator supercilii is the only muscle to draw the eyebrows medially
    B   The eybrows drain to the parotid and submandibular lymph nodes
    C   The superior palpebral sulcus is formed by orbicularis oculi
    D   In Caucasians, the lateral canthus lies 2 mm below the medial
    E   When blinking, the lids meet over the pupil

9 A True
  B False
  C True
  D False
  E True

Orbicularis oculi has fibres of levator palpebrae superioris crossing it. The palpebral portion of orbicularis inserts into the medial palpebral ligament and lateral palpebral raphe. The lacrimal portion lies posterior to the lacrimal sac causing it to dilate when blinking occurs. Part of orbucularis ensures apposition of the lower lid to the globe, and the glands of Moll separate the ciliary and palpebral portions.

10 A False
  B True
  C False
  D False
  E False

The orbital portion of orbicularis oculi and corrugator supercili draw the eyebrows medially. Like all orbital structures, the eyebrow's lymphatics drain to the submandibular and parotid nodes. The superior palpebral sulcus is formed by the insertion of fibres of levator palpebrae superioris into the skin, dividing the upper lid into orbital and tarsal portions. In Caucasians, the lateral canthus lies ≈2 mm above the medial, whereas in Orientals it lies some 3 mm higher still. The eyelids meet over the inferior cornea when blinking occurs.

11 The conjunctiva is innervated by branches of

A   The ciliary ganglion

B   The nasociliary nerve

C   Three nerves which traverse the superior orbital fissure

D   A nerve that originally conveys autonomic fibres from the pterygopalatine ganglion

E   A nerve innervating the cheek

12 Which of the following statements is/are correct?

A   The posterior conjunctival and anterior ciliary arteries anastomose 4 mm from the limbus

B   The conjunctival lymphatics drain to the lids

C   The superior tarsal conjunctiva is smooth and unindented

D   Equal numbers of lashes are present on each eyelid

E   The lashes are replaced after about 80 days

11 A False
    B True
    C True
    D True
    E True

The conjunctiva is innervated as follows:

Bulbar conjunctiva   – long ciliary nerves (nasociliary nerve)
Superior palpebral and – frontal and lacrimal nerves (V_1)
forniceal conjunctiva
Inferior palpebral and – infraorbital nerve (V_2, medially) lacrimal
forniceal conjunctiva   nerve (V_1, laterally)

The lacrimal, frontal and nasociliary nerves cross the superior orbital fissure. The maxillary nerve conveys autonomic fibres from the pterygopalatine ganglion and becomes the infraorbital nerve which supplies the cheek.

12 A False
    B True
    C True
    D False
    E False

The anterior and posterior conjunctival arteries anastomose with one another. The anterior conjunctival vessels are branches of the anterior ciliary arteries formed 4 mm from the limbus. The conjunctival lymphatics consist of a superficial and deep plexus which drain to the lymphatics vessels of the lids. The area of superior palpebral conjunctiva above the tarsal plate has horizontal folds due in part to the adjacent superior tarsal muscle. It also contains some elevations formed by Stieda's grooves, a number of small grooves in the conjunctiva. The lashes are arranged in two or three rows, with approximately 150 lashes in the upper lid and half that number in the lower. The lashes are shed every 4–5 months.

13 Which of the following statements about the conjunctiva is/are correct?

A   The lower lid's conjunctiva is completely adherent to the tarsal plate

B   The lateral fornix ends anterior to the equator

C   The conjunctiva is continuous with the corneal epithelium

D   Goblet cells are localized to the forniceal and bulbar conjunctiva

E   It contains numerous melanocytes in Caucasians

14 Which of the following statements regarding the precorneal tear film and its drainage is/are correct?

A   Mucin secreted by the tarsal glands prevents tears overflowing the lids

B   One-quarter of the aqueous layer is derived from the accessory lacrimal glands of Krause and Wolfring

C   Secretions of conjunctival goblet cells stabilize the tear film

D   More than 80% of the tears pass through the lower puncta

E   Blinking causes compression of the lacrimal sac

13 A False
 B False
 C True
 D False
 E True

Whereas the superior tarsal conjunctiva is completely adherent to the tarsal plate, only half of the inferior tarsal conjunctiva is so attached. The lateral fornix extends 14 mm from the limbus and therefore ends posterior to the equator. The conjunctival and corneal epithelia are continuous and meet at the limbus. The goblet cells mainly secrete mucin and are found throughout the conjunctiva, including the plica semilunaris. Melanocytes are present in the conjunctiva of all races, although they are unpigmented in Caucasians.

14 A False
 B False
 C True
 D False
 E False

The precorneal tear film consists of three layers: an inner mucinous, a middle aqueous and an outer lipid layer. The mucin secreted by the conjunctival goblet cells makes the corneal epithelium hydrophilic, helping to stabilize the tear film. Ninety-five per cent of the aqueous layer is derived from the lacrimal gland, with the remainder produced by the accessory lacrimal glands of Krause and Wolfring. The functions of the lipid layer, secreted by the Meibomian or tarsal glands, include preventing the tears overflowing the lid margin. Blinking causes contraction of the lacrimal portion of orbicularis, which dilates the lacrimal sac, drawing tears into the lacrimal drainage system. More than 50% of these tears pass through the upper punctum.

15 All the recti muscles
    A   Arise just from the common tendinous ring
    B   Are innervated on their conal surface by nerves that cross the superior orbital fissure
    C   Have Tenon's capsule reflected around them
    D   Have similar tendon lengths
    E   Insert anterior to the equator

16 Which of the following statements is/are correct?
    A   The orbital visual axes are parallel
    B   The common tendinous ring encircles part of both orbital fissures
    C   Superior rectus is the largest extraocular muscle
    D   Medial rectus inserts closest to the limbus
    E   The extraocular muscles all insert anterior to the equator

15 A False
  B True
  C True
  D False
  E True

The common tendinous ring is a fibrous ring, from which the four recti originate. Lateral rectus also attaches to a spine on the greater wing of the sphenoid, while superior and medial rectus attach to the dura of the optic nerve. The recti are innervated on their conal surface by III and VI, which enter the orbit through the superior orbital fissure within the common tendinous ring. Tenon's is reflected around all six extraocular muscles. The reflections around medial and lateral rectus form named check ligaments, while those around superior and inferior rectus help co-ordinate eyelid movements with those of the globe. The tendon lengths of the recti vary (from 3.7 mm to 8.8 mm) and they all insert anterior to the equator.

16 A False
  B False
  C False
  D True
  E False

The orbital axes form an angle of 23° to the globe's anteroposterior axis and an angle of 46° to one another. The common tendinous ring encircles the optic foramen and the medial end of the superior orbital fissure. Medial rectus is the largest muscle (although superior rectus is longer) and its inserts closest to the limbus, just 5.5 mm from the cornea. Although the four recti insert anterior to the equator, superior and inferior oblique insert into the posterosuperolateral and posteroinferolateral quadrants of the globe, respectively.

17 The fibres of superior rectus differ from those of procerus in

A Being shorter

B Running most of the length of the muscle

C Having a richer neurovascular supply

D Possessing three different types of end-plate

E Containing less elastic tissue

18 Lateral rectus

A Is stronger than its antagonist

B Is supplied by the lacrimal artery

C Is related superiorly to the lacrimal nerve

D Is a pure abductor in all positions of gaze

E At the orbital apex has VI lying between it and the optic nerve

17 A False
    B True
    C True
    D False
    E False

All the extraocular muscle fibres run almost the entire length of the muscle. Those of superior rectus, which is 42 mm long, are considerably longer than those of procerus. The extraocular muscle fibres have an extremely rich neural (and vascular) supply, with each motor neuron supplying only a few fibres. The fibres are surrounded by connective tissue with a high elastic content. There appear to be two types of motor end-plates, the classical type found in the thicker fast-contracting fibres and the *en grappe* end-plate of thin slow contracting ones.

18 A False
    B True
    C True
    D False
    E True

Lateral rectus is smaller and therefore weaker than its antagonist (medial rectus is the largest extraocular muscle). The lacrimal nerve and artery run along lateral rectus's upper border and supply it with a muscular arterial branch. In the primary position, lateral rectus functions as a pure abductor. In other positions of gaze, due to acting at an angle of 23° to the globe, it will have secondary actions of elevation or depression. At the orbital apex, the ciliary ganglion, VI and the ophthalmic artery all lie between lateral rectus and the optic nerve.

19 Superior oblique
   A   Arises from the body of the sphenoid superomedial to the optic foramen
   B   Acts at a similar angle to that of inferior oblique
   C   Is innervated by IV on its conal surface
   D   Acts in the primary position to depress, abduct and extort the globe
   E   When the globe is adducted 54°, it acts as a pure depressor

20 Inferior oblique
   A   Arises from the maxilla
   B   Passes superior to inferior rectus
   C   Is supplied by the division of III that conveys parasympathetic fibres
   D   Is only supplied by the ophthalmic artery
   E   Extorts the globe

21 Surgery to inferior oblique could damage the following
   A   Optic nerve
   B   Inferonasal vortex vein
   C   Ciliary ganglion
   D   Anterior ciliary arteries
   E   Fovea

19 A True
   B True
   C False
   D False
   E True

Superior oblique arises from the sphenoid superomedial to the optic foramen. Its tendon passes over the trochlea to act on the globe at an angle of $\approx 54°$, similar to the angle of action of inferior oblique (51°). It is supplied by IV on its upper surface and its actions in the primary position are depression, abduction and intorsion. When adducted nasally, its only action is depression.

20 A True
   B False
   C True
   D False
   E True

Inferior oblique arises from the orbital surface of the maxilla and passes posterolaterally beneath inferior rectus. It is innervated by the lower division of III, which conveys parasympathetic fibres to the ciliary ganglion. It is supplied by muscular branches from the ophthalmic and infraorbital arteries. Its primary action is elevation, but it also abducts and extorts the globe.

21 A True
   B False
   C True
   D False
   E True

Inferior oblique inserts 2 mm from the macula and it, the ciliary ganglion which is supplied by the nerve to inferior oblique, and the optic nerve may be damaged by traction on this muscle. The optic nerve lies only 5 mm from the insertion. The inferonasal vortex vein, which emerges on the other side of the globe to the insertion, is unlikely to be damaged by surgical manipulation. Likewise the anterior ciliary arteries, formed from the muscular branches to the four recti, will be similarly unaffected.

22 Which of the following statements is/are correct?
A Superior rectus elevates the globe maximally with the eye abducted
B Inferior oblique elevates the globe maximally with the eye adducted
C None of the extraocular muscles has non-bony origins
D Orbital fat extends from the orbital apex to the orbital septum
E Anterior to the common tendinous ring the four recti muscles have no attachments to one another

23 Which of the following muscles are principally responsible for looking at a fly landing on the end of one's nose?
A Left dilator pupillae
B Right superior oblique
C Left inferior oblique
D Right superior rectus
E Right and left medial recti

24 Muscle spindles
A Are more numerous in extraocular muscles than in trapezius
B Possess an afferent and efferent supply
C When passively stretched, relay via Ia fibres to cause intrafusal contraction
D Measure the force of muscle contraction
E Contain three main fibre types

22 A True
  B True
  C False
  D True
  E False
Due to superior rectus and inferior oblique acting at angles of 23° and 51°, they have their maximal effect with the globe abducted and adducted, respectively. Both superior and medial rectus are attached to the meninges of the optic nerve. Orbital fat extends from the orbital apex to the septum and fills part of the orbit left unfilled by other structures. An intermuscular membrane joins the sheaths of the four recti and is continuous with Tenon's capsule.

23 A False
  B True
  C False
  D False
  E True
Looking at the end of one's nose involves adduction, depression and accommodation. Some of the muscles involved in doing this are the medial recti, the superior obliques and the ciliary muscles.

24 A True
  B True
  C False
  D False
  E False
Muscle spindles (intrafusal fibres) monitor muscle length and the velocity of muscle contraction. They possess a motor (gamma efferent) and sensory (I alpha/II) supply and are much more numerous in muscles involved in precise actions. Stretching the muscle spindles triggers discharge from either the nuclear bag or nuclear chain fibres (depending on the nature of the stimulus) which, via I alpha neurons relaying to the anterior horn cells, causes extrafusal fibre (i.e. muscle) contraction.

25 **Which of the following statements about the four recti is/are correct?**

   A   Superior rectus has the shortest tendon

   B   Inferior rectus inserts furthest from the limbus

   C   Lateral rectus has the broadest tendon

   D   Medial rectus has the longest tendon

   E   Superior oblique passes above superior rectus to insert into the sclera

25 A False
B False
C False
D False
E False

Superior rectus has the broadest tendon (10.8 mm) and inserts furthest from the limbus (7.7 mm). Medial rectus possesses the shortest tendon, whereas lateral rectus has the longest. Superior oblique passes under the tendon of superior rectus, inserting in a fan-shaped manner in the posterosuperolateral scleral quadrant.

7 Cranial nerves and visual pathway

1 Which of the following statements regarding the origin and course of III is/are correct?

A It emerges as a single root from a nucleus lying level with the superior colliculus

B It leaves the brainstem after passing through the red nucleus

C It runs below and lateral to the free margin of the tentorium cerebelli

D It pierces the dura midway between the anterior and posterior clinoid processes

E Its branches cross the same part of the superior orbital fissure as VI

Cranial nerves and visual pathway: answers

1 A False
   B True
   C False
   D True
   E True

The oculomotor nerve, whose nucleus lies at the level of the superior colliculus, arises as a number of rootlets from the ventral surface of the midbrain, after crossing the red nucleus. It passes superomedial to the free margin of the tentorium and pierces the dura on the middle cranial fossa floor midway between the anterior and posterior clinoid processes. Both divisions of III pass through the superior orbital fissure, within the common tendinous ring, which is also traversed by the nasociliary and abducent nerves.

2 Regarding the distribution of fibres from III

    A   Levator palpebrae superioris only receives a motor supply from the superior division of III

    B   It innervates all the recti muscles at the junction of their middle and posterior thirds

    C   The parasympathetic supply to the iris is conveyed via the long ciliary nerves

    D   Superior rectus is innervated ipsilaterally

    E   Levator palpebrae superioris is bilaterally represented at the level of the oculomotor nuclei

3 Which of the following statements regarding III is/are correct?

    A   The parasympathetic fibres lie centrally in the precavernous sinus portion of the nerve

    B   A third nerve palsy causes the eye to remain in the primary position

    C   Accommodation is unaffected by such a palsy

    D   Compression of the nerve causes a partial ptosis

    E   The Edinger–Westphal nucleus lies ventral to the main oculomotor nucleus

2 A False
   B True
   C False
   D False
   E True

Levator palpebrae superioris has a double innervation. Its unstriated superior tarsal muscle is supplied by postganglionic sympathetic fibres from the superior cervical ganglion. These fibres are conveyed to the muscle by the upper division of III, which also supplies the larger striated component with motor fibres. III innervates all four recti muscles on their conal surface at the junction of their middle and posterior thirds. Parasympathetic fibres, derived from the Edinger–Westphal nucleus, are conveyed by the inferior division of III and the nerve to inferior oblique to the ciliary ganglion, where they synapse. The postganglionic fibres reach the iris and ciliary body via the short ciliary nerves. Superior rectus is innervated by the contralateral third nerve nucleus, while levator palpebrae superioris is supplied by both nuclei.

3 A False
   B False
   C False
   D False
   E False

Parasympathetic (pupillary) fibres lie peripherally in the proximal part of III. A complete oculomotor palsy results in the unopposed action of lateral rectus and superior oblique, with the eye looking down and out. Such a palsy, by interrupting the parasympathetic supply to the ciliary muscle, prevents accommodation. It also causes a complete ptosis by interrupting the motor supply to the striated part of levator palpebrae superioris and, depending on the location of the lesion, to the superior tarsal muscle as well. The accessory oculomotor (or Edinger–Westphal) nuclei lie posterior to the main oculomotor nuclei.

4 **The trochlear nerve**
   A   Is the only motor nerve to leave the brainstem dorsally
   B   Emerges from the brainstem at the level of the inferior colliculus
   C   Passes between two arteries like III
   D   Lies above III during part of its course
   E   Innervates superior oblique on its inferior surface

5 **Which of the following statements is/are correct?**
   A   The trochlear nucleus lies dorsal to the aqueduct
   B   Ablation of the right trochlear nucleus weakens intorsion of the right eye
   C   The trochlear nucleus is connected to the medial longitudinal fasciculus by a 7 mm long bundle of fibres
   D   The trochlear nerve lies close to the superior medullary velum
   E   A fourth nerve palsy interferes with upgaze

6 **The abducens nerve**
   A   Arises from the medulla
   B   Passes under the petrosphenoidal ligament
   C   May cross two venous sinuses in its course
   D   Enters the orbit between the two divisions of III
   E   May be damaged by raised intracranial pressure

4 A True
    B False
    C True
    D True
    E False

IV, whose nucleus lies at the level of the inferior colliculus, is the only motor cranial nerve to decussate and leave the brainstem dorsally. It emerges below the inferior colliculus and winds around the cerebral peduncle before passing between the posterior cerebral and superior cerebellar arteries, lateral to III. IV lies above III at the end of the cavernous sinus and innervates superior oblique on its upper surface.

5 A False
    B False
    C False
    D False
    E False

The nuclei of IV lie ventral to the aqueduct and, because the nerve decussates in the superior medullary velum, superior oblique is contralaterally innervated. The nuclei lie adjacent to the medial longitudinal fasciculus. Superior oblique's actions are to abduct, depress and intort the globe.

6 A False
    B True
    C True
    D True
    E True

VI emerges as a series of rootlets between the pons and the medulla. It passes under the petrosphenoidal ligament, entering the cavernous sinus often after crossing the inferior petrosal sinus. It then passes through the superior orbital fissure, within the common tendinous ring, lying between the two divisions of III. The nerve's course over the edge of the petrous temporal bone makes it liable to damage from elevated intracranial pressure which can cause coning.

7 **The abducens nerve nucleus**
   A Lies ventral to the genu of VII
   B Communicates indirectly with the nucleus of III
   C Sends fibres through Dorello's canal
   D Innervates lateral rectus on its extraconal surface
   E Supplies fibres which are unaffected by a basal skull fracture

8 **The relations of the trigeminal ganglion include**
   A Medially   – internal carotid artery
   B Laterally   – middle meningeal artery
   C Superiorly – uncus
   D Inferiorly – internal carotid artery
   E Anteriorly – temporal lobe

7 A True
   B True
   C True
   D False
   E False

The nucleus of VI lies ventral to the genu of VII, which forms the facial colliculus. It communicates with III, IV and VIII via the medial longitudinal fasciculus. Dorello's canal, through which VI passes, is formed by the petroclinoid ligament. Lateral rectus, like all the recti, is innervated on its conal surface at the junction of its middle and posterior thirds. Due to its close relationship to the skull base, VI is often damaged in basal skull fractures.

8 A True
   B True
   C True
   D True
   E True

The relations of the trigeminal ganglion are:

Medially   – cavernous sinus, internal carotid, III, IV and VI
Laterally – foramen spinosum transmitting the middle meningeal artery
Superiorly – uncus and temporal lobe
Inferiorly – internal carotid, motor root of V, greater and lesser petrosal nerves
Anteriorly – temporal lobe

9 **The trigeminal ganglion communicates with**
   A   The motor root of V
   B   Fibres surrounding the internal carotid artery
   C   Proprioceptive fibres from buccinator
   D   The maxillary sinus
   E   The scalp overlying the parietal bones

10 **Which of the following statements about the trigeminal nerve and ganglion is/are correct?**
   A   The smaller motor root emerges above the sensory root
   B   These two roots fuse at the trigeminal ganglion
   C   The ganglion lies lateral to the internal acoustic meatus
   D   The ganglion lies within a covering formed from arachnoid and pia
   E   The whole ganglion is bathed in cerebrospinal fluid

9 A False
 B True
 C True
 D True
 E True

The trigeminal ganglion has no connection with the motor root. V_1, V_2 and V_3 emerge from the ganglion's anterior border. Since the scalp overlying the frontal bones is supplied by V_1, and the maxillary sinus and proprioceptive supply to buccinator are innervated by V_2, all these structures communicate with the trigeminal ganglion. In addition, the ganglion receives a branch from the sympathetic plexus around the internal carotid artery.

10 A True
 B False
 C False
 D False
 E False

The smaller motor root lies above the sensory and only the latter root is attached to the trigeminal (Gasserian) ganglion. The ganglion lies medial to the internal acoustic meatus and its posterior half is enclosed by a sheath of dura that forms the trigeminal (Meckel's) cave. Since the dura is lined with arachnoid, only this half of the ganglion is bathed in cerebrospinal fluid.

11 The trigeminal nerve nuclei
  A Are five in number
  B Have the mesencephalic nucleus lying furthest medially
  C Consist of cell bodies of second-order neurons
  D Have a novel arrangement of their pain fibres
  E Communicate with the thalamus via uncrossed fibres in the spinal lemniscus

12 The maxillary nerve
  A Traverses the wall of the cavernous sinus and the foramen ovale
  B Supplies the dura of the anterior cranial fossa floor
  C Receives fibres from the inferior salivatory nucleus
  D Has branches accompanied by those of the third part of the maxillary artery
  E Innervates all the teeth of the upper jaw

11 A False
    B False
    C False
    D True
    E False

There are four trigeminal nerve nuclei – three sensory and one motor. The sensory nuclei (mesencephalic, main sensory and spinal) lie in continuity with one another and the motor nucleus lies furthest medially. The mesencephalic consists of the cell bodies of first-order neurons. Sensory fibres conveying pain and temperature to the spinal nucleus project as follows: V_1 inferiorly to nucleus caudalis, V_2 to nucleus interpolaris and V_3 superiorly to nucleus oralis. The trigeminal nerve nuclei communicate with the thalamus via the trigeminal lemniscus which predominantly consists of crossed fibres.

12 A False
    B False
    C False
    D True
    E True

V_2 runs in the wall of the cavernous sinus and passes through the foramen rotundum. Its meningeal branch (the middle meningeal nerve) innervates half of the middle cranial fossa floor, with the remainder supplied by nervus spinosus (the meningeal branch of V_3). Autonomic fibres from the inferior salivatory nucleus (of IX) are conveyed via the otic ganglion to the parotid gland. Branches of V_2, such as the posterior superior alveolar nerve, are accompanied by branches of the third part of the maxillary artery. The superior alveolar nerves supply the teeth of the upper jaw.

13 **The mandibular nerve**
    A   Is the only division of V to carry both sensory and motor fibres
    B   Supplies two autonomic ganglia
    C   Has a branch crossing the pterion
    D   Innervates the temporomandibular joint
    E   Innervates all the named salivary glands

14 **The following nerves pass through the middle ear**
    A   Tympanic branch of IX
    B   Greater petrosal nerve
    C   Lesser petrosal nerve
    D   VII
    E   Chorda tympani

13 A True
   B True
   C True
   D True
   E True

Whereas V_1 and V_2 are purely sensory, V_3 carries both motor (to the muscles of mastication) and sensory fibres. V_3 supplies the submandibular and otic ganglia which are attached to the lingual nerve and nerve to medial pterygoid, respectively. Nervus spinosus (the meningeal branch of V_3) accompanies the middle meningeal artery and its subsequent divisions, the anterior one of which crosses the pterion. The auriculotemporal nerve supplies articular branches to the temperomandibular joint as well as supplying the parotid gland. The lingual nerve supplies both the submandibular and sublingual glands.

14 A True
   B False
   C True
   D False
   E True

The tympanic branch of IX (Jacobson's nerve) enters the middle ear via the tympanic canaliculus and passes to the tympanic plexus where the lesser petrosal nerve arises. The latter nerve conveys parasympathetic fibres to the otic ganglion, where they synapse, before passing to the parotid gland in the auticulotemporal nerve. The chorda tympani leaves VII 6 mm above the stylomastoid foramen, entering the middle ear cavity via the posterior canaliculus. After crossing medial to the handle of the malleus, it leaves via the anterior canaliculus, emerging from the petrotympanic fissue, and joins the lingual nerve 2 cm below the skull base. VII has a complex course through a canal in the petrous temporal bone, but neither it, nor the greater petrosal nerve which arises from the geniculate ganglion, cross the middle ear cavity.

15 Cranial nerves, their roots or branches pass through the following
   A   Petrosal foramen
   B   Pterygoid canal
   C   Foramen spinosum
   D   Condylar canal
   E   Foramen magnum

16 Part or all of the following cranial nerve nuclei lie in the pons
   A   IV
   B   V
   C   VIII
   D   IX
   E   X

15 A False
    B True
    C True
    D False
    E True
The petrosal foramen does not exist. The nerve of the pterygoid canal is formed by the greater (derived from the geniculate ganglion) and deep petrosal nerves. The foramen spinosum transmits the middle meningeal artery and the meningeal branch of the mandibular nerve. The condylar canal is not always present and transmits an emissary vein from the sigmoid sinus. The spinal root of XI traverses the foramen magnum.

16 A False
    B True
    C True
    D True
    E False
The nucleus of IV lies in the midbrain at the level of the inferior colliculus. Part or all of the nuclei of V–IX lie in the pons. The trigeminal motor nucleus lies in the pons whereas the sensory nuclei extend throughout the midbrain. The nuclei of VIII lie at the pontomedullary junction, with the vestibular nuclei particularly lying in both the medulla and the pons. The inferior salivatory nucleus of IX lies in the pons. The vagal nuclei are found in the upper medulla.

17 The following arise at the pontomedullary junction
A   V
B   VII
C   IX
D   XII
E   Nervus intermedius

18 The following cranial nerves contain afferent fibres from Pascinian corpuscles
A   III
B   IV
C   V
D   VI
E   Spinal root of XI

19 The optic nerve
A   Is approximately 2 cm long
B   Is pierced inferomedially by the central retinal artery and vein
C   Is covered by dura intracranially
D   Becomes myelinated before crossing the lamina cribrosa and entering the orbit
E   Contains about 1.2 million third-order neuron axons

17 A False
B True
C False
D False
E True

The levels at which the cranial nerves emerge are as follows:

III	– superior colliculus
IV	– just below the inferior colliculus
V	– pons
VI, VII, VIII	– pontomedullary junction
IX–XII	– medulla

(Nervus intermedius emerges with VII.)

18 A False
B False
C True
D False
E False

Pascinian corpuscles are found predominantly in the skin. Fibres from them are thus only found in nerves with a cutaneous distribution, i.e. V.

19 A False
B True
C False
D False
E False

The optic nerve is approximately 4 cm long. Its 2.5 cm long intraorbital portion is pierced inferomedially 12 mm behind the globe by the central retinal artery and vein. Like all cranial nerves it has no dural covering intracranially and only becomes myelinated proximal to the lamina cribrosa. The optic nerve largely consists of the axons of 1.2 million ganglion cells which are second-order neurons.

20 **Which of the following statements about the optic nerve is/are correct?**
A   The posterior ciliary arteries supply the intraocular portion
B   The intraorbital portion receives a supply from the central retinal artery
C   The intracanalicular portion is supplied by a plexus derived from the ophthalmic artery
D   The optic disc's diameter is approximately 3 mm
E   The optic disc lies 6 mm medial to the fovea

21 **The optic nerve**
A   Intraorbitally is double its intraocular thickness
B   Is crossed inferiorly by the nerve to lateral rectus
C   Meets its fellow nerve between the internal carotid arteries
D   Receives fibres from the temporal retina that have an indirect course to the optic disc
E   Contains nasal retinal fibres that have an indirect course before decussating

20 A True
   B True
   C True
   D False
   E False

The intraocular portion of the optic nerve is supplied by the circle of Haller–Zinn, formed by branches of the posterior ciliary arteries. The intraorbital and intracanalicular portions are both supplied by a pial plexus from the ophthalmic artery. The intraorbital portion also receives a supply from central collateral branches of the central retinal artery. The optic disc is ≈ 1.5 mm in diameter and lies 3.4 mm medial to the fovea.

21 A True
   B False
   C True
   D True
   E True

Myelination increases the thickness of the optic nerve from 1.5 mm intraocularly to ≈ 3 mm intraorbitally. It is crossed superiorly by the nasociliary nerve and inferiorly by the nerve to medial rectus. The two intracranial optic nerves meet at the chiasm which lies between the internal carotid arteries. Fibres from the temporal retina pass around the macula and papillomacular bundle to reach the optic disc. Some nasal fibres loop in the ipsilateral optic tract or contralateral optic nerve (the anterior knee of Willibrand) before decussating.

22 Which of the following statements is/are correct?
A Macular fibres lie medially in the distal optic nerve
B Temporal macular fibres decussate anteriorly in the chiasm
C Nasal macular fibres decussate posteriorly in the chiasm
D Macular fibres lie superiorly in the optic tract
E In the lateral geniculate body, fibres conveying information from the peripheral retina lie posteriorly

23 The relations of the optic chiasm are
A Superiorly   – lumen of third ventricle
B Inferiorly   – sulcus chiasmaticus
C Anteriorly   – anterior communicating artery
D Posteriorly   – mamillary bodies
E Posterolaterally – optic tracts

22 A False
   B False
   C False
   D True
   E False

Macular fibres lie laterally in the distal optic nerve and adopt a central position as they approach the chiasm. Nasal macular fibres decussate centrally in the chiasm, although they may loop anteriorly or posteriorly prior to decussating. Temporal macular fibres do not of course decussate. In the optic tract, macular fibres lie superiorly whereas in the lateral geniculate body, fibres supplied by peripheral retinal photoreceptors lie anteriorly.

23 A False
   B False
   C True
   D False
   E True

The anatomical relations of the optic chiasm are:

Superiorly	– lamina terminalis
Inferiorly	– pituitary and diaphragma sellae
Anteriorly	– anterior cerebral and anterior communicating arteries
Laterally	– internal carotid arteries
Posteriorly	– tuber cinereum (the mamillary bodies lie posterior to this)
Posterolaterally	– optic tracts

24 The following arteries supply the optic chiasm

A Internal carotid

B Inferior hypophyseal

C Anterior choroidal

D Posterior communicating

E Ophthalmic

25 Which of the following statements is/are correct?

A Macular fibres occupy one-third of the optic nerve

B Sectioning the right optic nerve adjacent to the chiasm only causes right visual field loss

C Sectioning the right optic tract may cause right temporal field loss

D Illuminating identical points on each retina causes adjacent lateral geniculate body cells to fire

E The occipital eye field lies in the peristriate area

24 A True
   B False
   C False
   D True
   E False
The vascular supply to the optic chiasm is from a pial plexus supplied by the following:

Direct branches of the internal carotid artery
Superior hypophyseal artery
Anterior cerebral artery
Anterior and posterior communicating arteries

25 A True
   B False
   C True
   D False
   E False
Macular fibres occupy one-third of the optic nerve, although the macula covers only approximately one-twentieth of the retina. Sectioning the optic nerve adjacent to the chiasm divides fibres in the anterior knee of Wilbrand, forming a so-called junctional scotoma in the left visual field. Likewise, sectioning the optic tract adjacent to the chiasm would divide fibres looping posteriorly in the tract prior to decussating, causing ipsilateral field loss. As contralateral and ipsilateral fibres pass to different laminae in the lateral geniculate body, adjacent cells would not be stimulated by the image mentioned in D. The occipital eye field lies in the secondary visual area (Brodmann's area 18 and 19).

26 Which of the following statements about the optic tracts is/are correct?

A   All fibres in its lateral root reach the lateral geniculate body

B   The smaller medial root forms the superior brachium

C   They lie medial to III

D   They are covered by parts of the temporal lobe

E   They are supplied by the middle cerebral artery

27 The lateral geniculate body

A   Lies on the postero-inferior surface of the thalamus

B   Consists of six layers of similarly sized cells

C   Has its layers numbered from its medial border

D   Receives ipsilateral fibres in layer 3

E   Is supplied by the anterior choroidal artery

26 A False
 B False
 C False
 D True
 E False

The optic tract consists of two roots, with the medial root containing supraoptic commissural fibres. While most of the lateral root's fibres reach the lateral geniculate body, the remainder leave the tract in the superior brachium. These reach the pretectal nuclei to be involved in the pupillary light reflexes. The optic tracts lie lateral to III and are covered by the uncus. Their vascular supply is derived from a pial plexus supplied by the anterior choroidal, posterior communicating and middle cerebral arteries.

27 A True
 B False
 C False
 D True
 E True

The lateral geniculate body (LGB) lies on the undersurface of the pulvinar of the thalamus and consists of six layers of cells described as either magnocellular or parvocellular according to their size. The layers are numbered from the hilum of the LGB to its crest. Contralateral fibres pass to layers 1, 4 and 6, whereas ipsilateral ones end in layers 2, 3 and 5. The LGB's vascular supply is derived from thalamogeniculate branches of the posterior cerebral and the anterior choroidal branch of the internal carotid, which also supplies the choroid plexus.

28 The right lateral geniculate body
  A Lies on the dorsal surface of the brainstem
  B Receives all the fibres entering the right optic tract
  C Receives information from the right temporal and left nasal hemifields
  D Contains many fewer cells than the number of optic nerve axons
  E Is connected to the superior colliculus

29 The geniculocalcarine tract
  A Only contains afferent fibres
  B Conveys visual information from the ipsilateral temporal hemifield
  C Contains fibres passing around the tip of the inferior horn of the lateral ventricle
  D An inferior homonomous quadrantanopia develops when damaged at the point referred to in (C)
  E Is solely supplied by the posterior cerebral arteries

28 A True
   B False
   C False
   D False
   E True

The lateral geniculate nuclei or bodies (LGB) lie on the dorsal surface of the brainstem (adjacent to the pulvinar of the thalamus). Some of the fibres in the optic tract leave prior to reaching the LGB, including those forming the brachium of the superior colliculus. The right LGB receives visual information from the right nasal and left temporal hemifields (right temporal and left nasal hemiretinae), with collateral and ipsilateral fibres passing to laminae 1, 4 and 6 and 2, 3 and 5, respectively. Each LGB contains about 1 000 000 cells, approximately the same as the number of axons in the optic nerve.

29 A False
   B False
   C True
   D False
   E False

The geniculocalcarine tracts (optic radiations) contain both afferent and efferent fibres and convey information from the ipsilateral temporal (nasal hemifield) and contralateral nasal hemiretinae. Some of the fibres pass around the tip of the inferior horn of the lateral ventricle forming Meyer's loop. Damage to the radiation at this point results in a superior homonomous quadrantanopia. The vascular supply to the radiation consists of branches of the anterior choroidal, middle cerebral and posterior cerebral arteries.

30 The calcarine sulcus

   A   In part lies adjacent to the corpus callosum

   B   Is limited laterally by the lunate sulcus

   C   Is separated from the parieto-occipital sulcus by the cuneate gyrus

   D   Is about 0.5 cm deep

   E   Has fibres from the upper retinal quadrants passing to its inferior lip

31 The visual cortex

   A   Lies along the lower lip of the anterior part of the calcarine sulcus

   B   Extends along both lips of the posterior part

   C   Does not extend onto the lateral hemispheric surface

   D   Has a characteristic cross-sectional appearance

   E   May be supplied by branches of the internal carotid and vertebral arteries

30 A True
  B True
  C True
  D False
  E False

The calcarine sulcus runs from the middle of the lunate sulcus to end close to the splenium of the corpus callosum. The cuneate gyrus separates the calcarine and parieto-occipital sulci, although superficial inspection would suggest that the two sulci are continuous. The calcarine sulcus is particularly deep, producing an indentation in the posterior horn of the lateral ventricle (calcar avis). Fibres from the superior retinal quadrants (inferior visual field) pass to the superior part of the wall of the calcarine sulcus.

31 A True
  B True
  C False
  D True
  E False

The visual cortex (Brodmann's areas 17, 18 and 19) lies along the inferior lip of the anterior part of the calcarine sulcus, both lips of the posterior part and extends as far as the lunate sulcus on the lateral hemispheric surface. It contains the striate cortex named after the stria of Gennari, a white line in the fourth cortical layer formed in part by myelinated optic radiation and intracortical connecting fibres. The visual cortex is supplied by both the posterior cerebral (a branch of the basilar) and middle cerebral (a branch of the internal carotid) arteries.

32   The primary visual area (area 17)

A   Lies only on the medial surface of the occipital lobe

B   Possesses a stria partly formed by myelinated optic radiation fibres

C   The stria mentioned in B lies in an expanded cortical layer

D   Has a surface area of some 3 cm^2

E   Is connected indirectly to the contralateral striate cortex

33   Regarding the primary visual area (area 17)

A   It consists of six laminae (layers)

B   It has a smaller lamina III than the motor cortex

C   Only cells in its lamina II project to areas 18 and 19

D   Its lamina V projects to the area for visual memory

E   Its lamina VI projects to the occipital eye field

32 A False
 B True
 C True
 D False
 E True

The primary visual area (area 17) extends onto the lateral hemispheric surface and contains the stria of Gennari. It is formed by an enlarged cortical lamina (lamina IV), consisting in part of myelinated optic radiation fibres. The primary visual cortex has an approximate surface area of 30 cm^2 and communicates with its fellow via the secondary visual area.

33 A True
 B True
 C False
 D False
 E False

The primary visual area (area 17) consists of six laminae, like other cortical areas. It differs from them in having a thin lamina III and a greatly expanded lamina IV. Cells in both lamina II and III project to the secondary visual areas (18 and 19). Lamina V projects to the superior colliculus, while lamina VI projects to the lateral geniculate body.

8 Ocular anatomy

1 Regarding the globe
    A   The anterior segment lies anterior to the plane of the iris
    B   The optic axis joins the fovea with the anterior pole
    C   The globe has equal horizontal and vertical diameters
    D   The axial length is decreased in short-sightedness
    E   It lies closer to the orbital roof than floor

2 The cornea
    A   Is circular in shape
    B   Is thickest centrally
    C   Is innervated by a single plexus derived from V_1
    D   Has a multilayered squamous epithelium
    E   Contains three acellular layers

Ocular anatomy: answers

1 A False
   B False
   C False
   D False
   E True

The globe consists of two segments. The anterior segment contains the anterior and posterior chambers (between the cornea and iris, and iris and lens, respectively). The posterior segment represents the area posterior to the lens. The optic axis connects the eye's anterior and posterior poles, while the visual axis connects the foveola with the nodal point. The globe's vertical diameter (23 mm) is less than its horizontal (23.5 mm), while its axial length is increased in most myopes (short-sighted individuals). It lies closer to the roof than the floor.

2 A False
   B False
   C False
   D True
   E False

The cornea is an ellipse, with horizontal and vertical diameters of 11.7 mm and 10.6 mm, respectively. It is thinnest centrally (0.6 mm), increasing to 1.2 mm peripherally. It contains three nerve plexuses (annular, subepithelial and intra-epithelial) all derived from V_1. The epithelium comprises 5–6 layers of non-keratinized squamous cells. The two acellular layers present are Bowman's and Descemet's membranes. The corneal stroma contains numerous fibroblasts interspersed among the tightly packed collagen fibres.

3 The corneal stroma

   A   Forms 70% of the corneal thickness

   B   Consists of highly ordered lamellae 2 nm thick

   C   Is the strongest corneal layer

   D   Blends with sclera peripherally

   E   Possesses a fine lymphatic network

4 Which of the following statements is/are correct?

   A   The corneal epithelium has a smooth outer surface

   B   It regenerates from central stem cells if damaged

   C   The corneal epithelium's deepest cells are attached to Descemets's membrane by desmosomes

   D   The corneal endothelium consists of a single layer of polygonal cells

   E   This endothelium is unable to regenerate in humans

3 A False
   B False
   C False
   D True
   E False

The corneal stroma consists of 200–250 lamellae of highly ordered collagen fibres, with each lamella orientated at 90° to the one above. The lamellae are ≈ 2 μm thick and the corneal stroma accounts for $\approx 90\%$ of the corneal thickness. Descemet's membrane, despite its comparative thinness (only 10 μm) is the strongest corneal layer. At the limbus the regular arrangement of corneal fibres blends directly with the irregular arrangement of the scleral ones. In order to maintain its transparency, the cornea is avascular and has no lymphatic vessels.

4 A False
   B False
   C False
   D True
   E True

The outermost corneal epithelial cells possess both microplicae and microvilli. Regeneration of epithelial cells occurs from stem cell lying at the limbus in folds called the pallisades of Vogt. The deepest columnar cells of the epithelium are attached to a basal lamina by hemidesmosomes and this lamina in turn is attached to Bowman's layer. The human corneal endothelium consists of polygonal cells, incapable of regeneration.

5 Tenon's capsule

    A   Sheathes the globe up to the posterior border of the limbus

    B   Lies in contact with orbital fat

    C   Is pierced by all the ciliary vessels and nerves

    D   Is reflected around all the muscles that move the globe

    E   Supports the globe

6 The sclera

    A   Has ciliary muscle attached to it

    B   Is firmly attached to overlying Tenon's capsule

    C   Is supplied by three sets of ciliary arteries

    D   Is thickest at the sites of muscle insertion

    E   Is grooved on its innermost surface

5 A False
  B True
  C False
  D True
  E True

Tenon's capsule extends from an insertion 1.5 mm behind the limbus to blend with the meninges around the optic nerve, and posteriorly is in contact with orbital fat. At other points it is loosely attached to the episclera (the outermost scleral layer), creating a potential episcleral space. Although it is pierced by the posterior ciliary vessels and nerves, the anterior ciliary arteries derived from the muscular branches of the ophthalmic do not cross it. Tenon's capsule is reflected around the extraocular muscles, forming prominent check ligaments in the case of medial and lateral rectus. These, together with an inferior thickening of Tenon's, the suspensory ligament of Lockwood, serve to support the globe.

6 A True
  B False
  C True
  D False
  E True

The scleral spur is a scleral projection lying behind Schlemm's canal, to which the ciliary muscle attaches. The episclera, the outermost scleral layer, is only loosely attached to Tenon's capsule. The sclera posterior to the equator is supplied by the long and short posterior ciliary arteries, while the anterior ciliary arteries supply the episclera. The thickness of the sclera varies considerably from ≈ 1 mm posteriorly to ≈ 0.6 mm at the equator and a mere 0.3 mm behind the insertions of the four recti. The innermost scleral layer (lamina fusca) is grooved by the long ciliary vessels and nerves passing in the perichoroidal space between it and the choroid.

7 Which of the following statements about the limbal area is/are correct?
  A   It is 1.5–2 mm wide
  B   It is the site where the cornea and sclera merge
  C   The conjunctival and corneal epithelia meet here
  D   Tenon's capsule fuses with the episclera at this point
  E   It is crossed by unmyelinated fibres innervating the cornea

8 The canal of Schlemm
  A   Is a channel of constant width encircling the globe
  B   Lies posterior to the scleral spur
  C   Drains by 25–30 collector channels
  D   Eventually drains to the major venous circle of the iris
  E   Is bypassed by the aqueous veins (of Ascher)

7 A True
    B True
    C True
    D False
    E False

The 1.5–2 mm wide limbus is the site of the corneoscleral junction. The corneal epithelium becomes continuous with that of the conjunctiva, while Bowman's layer becomes the conjunctival lamina propria. Tenon's capsule is fused tightly to the sclera 1.5 mm posterior to the limbus. Some 60–80 nerves cross the limbus, losing their myelin sheaths after penetrating several millimetres into the cornea.

8 A False
    B False
    C True
    D False
    E False

Schlemm's canal is an endothelial lined channel encircling the globe. It runs either as a single channel or as multiple branches that subsequently reunite to form a main channel. Its width therefore varies along its course. It lies anterior to the scleral spur, draining via 25–30 collector channels into three venous plexuses (deep scleral, intrascleral and episcleral) and then into the anterior ciliary veins. No major venous circle of the iris exists. The aqueous veins of Ascher are collector channels that bypass the deep scleral plexus and drain instead into conjunctival veins.

9   The iris
   A   At its pupillary margin lies ≈ 2 mm from the anterior capsule of the lens
   B   Is thickest at the ciliary margin
   C   Has Fuch's crypts within the epithelium
   D   Contains an annulus of muscle that contracts during accommodation
   E   Has the major arterial circle lying within it

10   The ciliary body
   A   Is the same colour as the choroid
   B   Has the pars plicata lying adjacent to the retina
   C   Is innervated by fibres from the nerve to inferior oblique
   D   Has longitudinal (meridional) muscle fibres lying anteriorly
   E   Has two epithelial layers whose cells lie with the apex of the one adjacent to the base of the other

9 A False
   B False
   C False
   D True
   E False

The iris's pupillary margin lies in contact with the anterior capsule of the lens. The iris is thickest at the collarette ≈1.6 mm from the pupillary margin and thinnest at the iris root (ciliary margin). Fuchs' crypts are crypts in the iris stroma visible on the anterior iris surface. Sphincter pupillae is a band of muscle some 1 mm thick arranged around the pupillary margin and causes pupillary constriction to occur when the eye accommodates. The major arterial circle of the iris lies in the ciliary body anterior to the circular ciliary muscle fibres. It is formed by an anastomosis between the seven anterior and the two long posterior ciliary arteries.

10 A False
    B False
    C True
    D False
    E False

The ciliary body is covered by two layers of epithelial cells lying apex to apex. The pigmented outer layer makes the ciliary body black, whereas the choroid is brown. The ciliary body contains some 70 ciliary processes. This region of the choroid is the pars plicata, while the pars plana lies adjacent to the ora serrata. Parasympathetic fibres conveyed to the ciliary ganglion by the nerve to inferior oblique reach the ciliary muscle in the short ciliary nerves. The muscle consists of circular, longitudinal (meridional) and oblique fibres. The longitudinal fibres predominantly attach to the scleral spur, while the circular fibres lie most anteriorly.

11 The lens
A   Is a symmetrical biconvex structure
B   Has a capsule that is thickest adjacent to the equator
C   Contains cells dividing maximally at the poles
D   Has an embryonic nucleus with an erect Y-shaped suture anteriorly
E   Contains elongated cells some 100 μm long

12 Which of the following occur during accommodation?
A   The anterior pole of the lens moves anteriorly
B   The lens diameter increases
C   The lens becomes thicker
D   The anterior pole of the lens becomes more convex
E   Sphincter pupillae contracts

11 A False
   B True
   C False
   D False
   E False

The lens is biconvex with the anterior surface curved less than the posterior. The radius of curvature is ≈ 10 mm anteriorly and ≈ 6 mm posteriorly. The lens capsule is 3–20 μm thick and thickest near the equator. Maximal division of epithelial cells to form new lens fibres occurs at the equator. The fetal nucleus forms Y-shaped suture lines with an erect suture anteriorly and an inverted suture posteriorly. The embryonic nucleus predates the fetal one and forms a central group of cells. The hexagonal lens fibres extend from (close to) one pole to the other and are some 8–12 mm long.

12 A True
   B False
   C True
   D True
   E True

Ciliary muscle contraction relaxes the tension on the lens zonule allowing the lens to adopt a more globular shape. This increases the refractive index of the lens, permitting the eye to focus on nearer objects. During accommodation the lens thickens; its diameter therefore decreases as the lens becomes more globular. Its anterior pole moves anteriorly as well as becoming more convex and the lens moves slightly inferiorly. In addition, both convergence and pupillary constriction occur.

13 **Which of the following statements is/are correct?**
   A   At rest the eye is focused at infinity
   B   Accommodation causes an increase in lens thickness
   C   The fibres of the lens zonule only connect the lens and ciliary processes
   D   The lens capsule is composed of a single layer of fibres
   E   A potential space exists between the posterior lens capsule and the anterior hyaloid face

14 **Which of the following statements about the vitreous is/are correct?**
   A   An embryological remnant of the primary vitreous is present in all young adult eyes
   B   Cloquet's canal communicates with the posterior vitreous base
   C   The tertiary vitreous forms a structure that is attached to the ciliary processes
   D   Wieger's ligament attaches to the lens ≈4 mm behind the equator
   E   Petit's canal lies between the lens and the anterior hyaloid face

13 A False
    B True
    C False
    D False
    E True

At rest the eye is focused at a distance of 1 m. Contraction of the ciliary muscle during accommodation relaxes the tension on the zonule, allowing the lens to thicken. The zonule connects not just the lens with the ciliary processes, as fibres run from the ora serrata to the lens as well as from one ciliary process to another. The lens capsule consists of some 40 lamellae each ≈ 40 nm thick. The potential retrolenticular space (of Berger) lies between the posterior lens capsule and the anterior hyaloid face.

14 A True
    B True
    C True
    D False
    E True

The primary vitreous, which is fully developed by nine weeks, subsequently regresses leaving Cloquet's canal as an embryological remnant in all eyes. This canal passes from the posterior margin of the membrana plicata to a glial adhesion around the disc (the posterior vitreous base/area of Martegiani). Other remnants may occasionally be present including Mittendorf's spot and persistent primary hyperplastic vitreous. The tertiary vitreous develops into the lens zonule which is attached to the ciliary processes, lens and ora serrata. Wieger's (hyaloideocapsular) ligament is the site of attachment of the anterior vitreous to the lens 1 mm behind the equator. Petit's canal (retrozonular space) is a small space between the lens zonule and the anterior vitreous.

15 **The choroid**
A Is thickest anteriorly
B Does not extend beyond the ora serrata
C Conveys a neurovascular supply to the front of the globe
D Has a capillary network densest at the posterior pole
E Nourishes the outermost part of the retina

16 **Which of the following statements about the retina is/are correct?**
A It contains ten times as many rods as cones
B It extends further anteriorly on its lateral than its medial side
C Its pigment epithelial cells have smooth basal surfaces
D The rod and cone cells are of similar length
E The cell bodies of the second-order neurons in the visual pathway are of uniform size

17 Which of the following statements is/are correct?

A   The retina is thickest at the ora serrata
B   The vitreous base is only attached to the pars plana
C   The volume of the posterior chamber is 0.6 ml
D   The trabecular meshwork is 0.2 mm wide
E   The precorneal tear film is 0.1 mm thick

18 The central retinal artery

A   Is larger than the central retinal vein
B   Is approximately 1 mm in diameter
C   Pierces the optic nerve 12 mm behind the globe
D   Is surrounded by just pia and arachnoid as it courses to the centre of the optic nerve
E   Never anastomoses with other vessels
F   Only supplies the retina
G   Supplies the retina up to its outer nuclear layer
H   Does not supply the macula

17 A False
   B False
   C False
   D False
   C False

The retina, which is thickest at the optic disc (0.56 mm) and thins anteriorly (0.1 mm at the ora serrata), is thinnest of all at the fovea (0.09 mm). The vitreous base is an area some 2 mm wide where the vitreous is firmly attached to the ora serrata and the pars plana. The volume of the anterior chamber is ≈ 0.2 ml, whereas that of the posterior chamber is 0.06 ml. The trabecular meshwork is 0.8–1 mm wide, while the precorneal tear film is ≈ 7 μm thick.

18 A False
   B False
   C True
   D False
   E False
   F False
   G False
   H False

The central retinal artery, like most arteries, is smaller than its accompanying vein. Approximately 0.28 mm in diameter, it pierces the dura and arachnoid of the optic nerve 12 mm behind the globe, acquiring a covering from each as well as from pia. Very small anastomoses do occur between the circle of Haller–Zinn and the central retinal artery, with 15–20% of people possessing a cilioretinal artery. Apart from supplying the inner two-thirds of the retina as far as the inner nuclear layer, the central retinal artery also supplies the pial covering of the nerve and, via its central collateral branch, fibres in the optic nerve.

9 Embryology

1 **In the 14–17 mm human embryo (≈6 weeks old), the following occur**
   A Optic chiasm forms
   B Retinal differentiation begins
   C Fetal fissure starts closing
   D Primary lens fibres form
   E Pigmentation of the retinal pigment epithelium begins

2 **In the 50 mm human embryo (≈10 weeks old), the following structures are already developed**
   A Secondary lens fibres
   B Ciliary muscle
   C Lens zonule
   D Tarsal glands
   E Myelinated optic nerve fibres

Embryology: answers

1   A   False
     B   True
     C   True
     D   True
     E   False

In the 6-week-old embryo, retinal differentiation begins, formation of primary lens fibres occurs and the fetal fissure starts closing (ending by the 17 mm stage). The optic chiasm forms at $7\frac{1}{2}$ weeks. Pigmentation of the retinal pigment epithelium begins at 6–7 mm (3 weeks) and is the first pigment to be deposited in the body.

2   A   False
     B   False
     C   False
     D   True
     E   False

The 10-week-old embryo has already developed tarsal glands. The lens zonule is derived from the tertiary vitreous at about the 60 mm stage, while the secondary lens fibres form at ≈ 70 mm and the ciliary muscle at ≈ 110 mm (4 months). Myelination of the optic nerve begins at 7 months and reaches the lamina cribrosa shortly before term.

3 Neural crest cells give rise to the following
   A Dorsal root ganglia of V, VII, IX and X
   B Dorsal root ganglia of III, IV and VI
   C Osteoblasts
   D Osteoclasts
   E Cartilage

4 The following are derived from surface ectoderm
   A Tarsal glands
   B Corneal stroma
   C Ciliary muscle
   D Lens
   E Sclera

5 The following are partially or completely derived from mesoderm
   A Descemet's membrane
   B Choroid
   C Iris smooth muscle
   D Ciliary body epithelium
   E Fascia bulbi

3 A True
   B False
   C False
   D False
   E True

Neural crest cells form the sensory ganglia (dorsal root ganglia) of both spinal and cranial nerves; hence of V, VII, IX and X, but not of the motor nerves III, IV and VI. They also form melanocytes, odontoblasts, meninges, Schwann cells, bone and cartilage.

4 A True
   B False
   C False
   D True
   E False

Surface ectoderm forms the epithelium of the cornea, conjunctiva and eyelids, as well as that of associated structures such as the tarsal and lacrimal glands.

5 A True
   B True
   C False
   D False
   E True

Mesoderm forms:

Orbital walls
Extraocular muscles
Tenon's capsule
Sclera
Choroid
Descemet's membrane, corneal stroma and endothelium
(Bowman's membrane is an anterior stromal condensation)
Iris stroma (+ anterior epithelium)

6 The following are derived from neutral ectoderm

  A Ganglion cells
  B Optic chiasm
  C Retinal pigment epithelium
  D Iris stroma
  E Müller cells

7 Which of the following statements about central nervous system development is/are correct?

  A The neural tube forms from the neural plate at the 3-week stage
  B The neural tube starts closing in the thoracic region
  C The cranial neuropore closes before the caudal one
  D The primary brain vesicles contain basal and alar plates
  E The corpora quadrigemina are derived from the mesencephalon

8 Which of the following statements about the pituitary gland is/are correct?

  A The pituitary is partially derived from ectoderm
  B Rathke's pouch only forms the adenohypophysis
  C The infundibulum forms both the pituitary stalk and posterior pituitary
  D The pituitary stalk is a completely solid structure
  E Enlarging pituitary tumours initially compress superonasal chiasmal fibres

6 A True
  B True
  C True
  D False
  E True
  Neural ectoderm forms:

  Retina and retinal pigment epithelium
  Sphincter and dilator pupillae
  Posterior pigment epithelium of the iris
  The neural portion of the optic nerve and chiasm

7 A True
  B False
  C True
  D True
  E True
  The neural tube is derived from the neural plate with fusion commencing in the cervical region. The cranial neuropore closes first, at the 18–20 somite stage (≈ 5 mm length embryo). The basal and alar plates are the motor and sensory areas of the primary brain vesicles. The four colliculi (corpora quadrigemina) are derived from the alar plates of the mesencephalon (midbrain).

8 A True
  B False
  C True
  D False
  E False
  The pituitary gland is derived from both ectoderm (Rathke's pouch) and the infundibulum (part of the diencephalon). Rathke's pouch forms the adenohypophysis (anterior lobe) and pars intermedia. The infundibulum forms the neurohypophysis (posterior lobe) and pituitary stalk, into which the infundibular recess extends for a variable distance. Enlarging pituitary tumours, with the exception of craniopharyngiomas, initially compress inferonasal chiasmal fibres.

9 **Which of the following statements about ocular development is/are correct?**

  A The cavity of the diencephalon communicates with that of the optic vesicle

  B Failure of optic cup closure leads to colobomata

  C The macula forms at the 5-month stage and is fully developed at term

  D The hyaloid arterial system carries no blood by the 7-month stage

  E Myelination of the optic nerve begins at the lamina cribrosa before term

10 **A full-term infant's eye differs from an adult's in having**

  A A smaller globe, some 12 mm in diameter

  B Less iris pigmentation

  C A narrower angle

  D A large pupil

  E Medial rectus inserting closer to the limbus

11 **Which of the following statements about the pharyngeal pouches is/are correct?**

  A They develop from surface ectoderm

  B The middle ear cavity forms from the proximal part of the first pouch

  C The palatine tonsil is derived from the second pouch

  D The parathyroid glands are formed from two adjacent pouches

  E The thyroid gland's calcitonin-secreting cells are derived from the fourth pouch

9 A True
   B False
   C False
   D True
   E False

The optic vesicle is an evagination of the forebrain and the two communicate, initially directly, and later via the optic stalk which arises from the diencephalon (part of the forebrain). Failure of closure of the choroidal fissure leads to colobomata of the iris, lens, choroid and retina. The macula lutea forms at 5 months, but is only fully developed several months after birth, partly explaining the poor central fixation of neonates. Myelination of the optic nerve begins at about 7 months centrally, extending distally to reach the lamina cribrosa shortly before term.

10 A False
    B True
    C True
    D False
    E True

A full-term infant's eye is smaller, at ≈ 14–16 mm, than an adult's and has more refractive media (especially the lens) to prevent excessive hypermetropia. Iris pigmentation commences a few days after birth and the infant irido corneal angle is narrower than that of adults. Infants possess a small pupil, and medial rectus inserts adjacent to the limbus.

11 A False
    B False
    C True
    D True
    E False

The pharyngeal pouches develop as outpouchings of the primitive foregut. The distal part of the first pouch forms the middle ear cavity, while the parathyroid glands form the third and fourth pouches. The fifth pouch forms the ultimobranchial body from which the thyroid's parafollicular or C cells are derived.

12 The following are derived from cartilage of the first pharyngeal arch
A   Thyroid cartilage
B   Malleus
C   Incus
D   Stapes
E   Arytenoid cartilage

13 The following are derived embryologically from the same pharyngeal arch as stylopharyngeus
A   Lesser horn of the hyoid bone
B   Greater horn of the hyoid bone
C   Part of the body of the hyoid bone
D   Stylohyoid ligament
E   Styloid process

14 The thyroid gland
A   Arises from the foramen caecum, at the junction of the anterior one-third and posterior two-thirds of the tongue
B   Becomes functional in the neonate
C   Remains connected to the tongue as it descends
D   Is supplied exclusively by branches of the external carotid and subclavian arteries
E   Is enclosed in pretracheal fascia

12 A False
   B True
   C True
   D False
   E False

The malleus and incus are derived from cartilage of the first pharyngeal arch. The stapes is formed from the second arch, while the thyroid and arytenoid cartilages are fourth-arch derivatives.

13 A False
   B True
   C True
   D False
   E False

Stylopharyngeus is derived from the third pharyngeal arch, together with the lower part of the body and greater horn of the hyoid bone. The lesser horn, styloid process and stylohyoid ligament are all second-arch derivatives.

14 A False
   B False
   C True
   D False
   E True

The thyroid gland arises at the foramen caecum, which lies at the junction of the anterior two-thirds and posterior third of the tongue. During its descent it is attached to the tongue by the thyroglossal duct and becomes functional at three months of gestation. Its vascular supply may include the thyroid ima artery, in addition to the superior and inferior thyroid vessels.

15 Regarding the ear's development
   A   The pinna is formed from the second pharyngeal cleft
   B   The middle ear is formed from part of the first pharyngeal cleft
   C   The otic placodes appear a the 3-week stage
   D   The semicircular canals develop as outpouchings from the saccule
   E   The hair cells are all covered by the tectorial membrane

15 A False
    B True
    C True
    D False
    E False

The pinna is derived from ≈ 6 mesenchymal hillocks. The semicircular canals are derived from outpouchings of part of the otic vesicle that forms the utricle. Only the outer hair cells are covered by the tectorial membrane.

Bibliography

Choosing textbooks is inevitably a personal choice, but I found the following particularly helpful:

Barr, M. L. and Kiernan, J. A. (1988) *The Human Nervous System*, Lippincott, Philadelphia.

McMinn, R. M. H. (1990) *Last's Anatomy*, Churchill Livingstone, Edinburgh.

Romanes, G. J. (1981) *Cunningham's Textbook of Anatomy*, Oxford University Press, London.

Sadler, T. W. (1985) *Langman's Medical Embryology*, Williams and Wilkins, Baltimore.

Snell, R. S. and Lemp, M. A. (1989) *Clinical Anatomy of the Eye*, Blackwell, Oxford.

Williams, P.L., Warwick, R., Dyson, M., Bannister, L.H. (eds) (1989) *Gray's Anatomy*, Churchill Livingstone, Edinburgh.

Wolff, E. (1976) *Anatomy of the Eye and Orbit*, H. K. Lewis, London.

Bibliography